The Dhance:

A Caregiver's Search for Meaning

By Coy F. Cross II, PhD

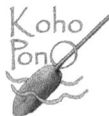

Koho
Pono

The Dhance: A Caregiver's Search for Meaning
Published by Koho Pono, LLC
Clackamas, Oregon USA
http://KohoPono.com

For general information on our other products, please contact
our Customer Service Department within the USA at 503-723-
7392 or visit *http://KohoPono.com*.

Cover art by Jain Martin, (c) 2012, *(Pen & Pencil, Photoshop,
Mixed Media)*

Soft cover edition 20may2012
Library of Congress Control Number: 2012938521
ISBN: 978-0-9845424-2-0

Manufactured in the United States of America

The Dhance

It is a dance which humanity agrees to dance with God—a dance undertaken without promise or hope; yet each person knows that the dance will end in unification.

- *Carol Ruth Knox, dissertation, page 192*

This book is a story of life at its best in the worst of experiences in the human journey. It gives us hope that we can always grow and discover who we truly are and what is important in life. A love story filled with life skills.

- Rev Beth Ann Suggs, PCC; Unity Minister

More than a powerful love story, The Dhance serves as a Spiritual Practice guide to courageously working through a major life crisis. Coy shares how being spiritually centered can help you avoid becoming overwhelmed by pain and loss while still remaining intensely present supporting a loved one with a life-threatening challenge. Learn how to love more deeply and to stay open to the spiritual lessons of life's difficult circumstances. I encourage you to read "The Dhance".

- Greg Finch, Licensed Teacher, Unity Worldwide Ministries

Respected historian, Doctor Coy F. Cross has written a much different book in "The Dhance". Cross has combined a long-time desire to write on the teachings of spiritual mentor, Carol Ruth Knox, and his family's reliance on those principles during his wife's life-threatening illness. The result is an amazing love story.

- Terence Docherty, teacher

"The Dhance" is a story of the search for deeper meaning within a loved one's serious illness. It also tells of a love that grows stronger as Coy and his wife Carol face their greatest challenge. Coy has written a beautiful account of using "practical spirituality" to deal with his wife's cancer and finding "God in this, too." I highly recommend this book to anyone facing a difficult life challenge or anyone looking for a great love story.

- Jim Lee, Unity Minister

Dedication

To the two Carols

Table of Contents

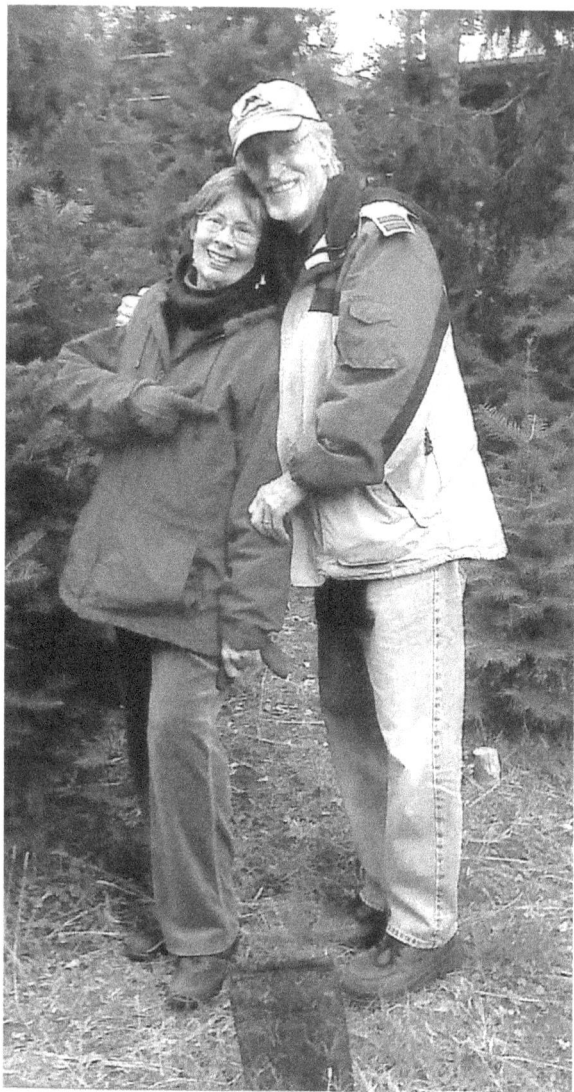

Coy and Carol Martha

Preface

This is not the book I intended to write. For more than twenty years I planned a book highlighting my friend Reverend Carol Ruth Knox's spiritual teachings. She opened my eyes to spiritual concepts that I had never before considered.

I struggled for years trying to understand her violent death at the hand of an intruder: a young, pregnant woman who killed herself as police closed in and whose motive or connection to Carol Ruth the police could never determine.

Eventually, I decided to use Carol Ruth's lessons in my attempt to understand her life and death. In preparation, I gathered every cassette tape and the few video recordings of her Sunday sermons and all her writings I could find, including her dissertation. Although I immersed myself in the material, the writing progressed slowly. A historian by profession, I found myself writing in the historian's detached style, as the observer, unaffected by the story. But I was affected by the events I wrote about. Carol Ruth was a close, personal friend, whom I loved dearly. So after more than two years of writing, I had completed just three chapters.

Carol Ruth's teachings took on added importance in May 2009 when my wife, also named Carol, was diagnosed with ovarian cancer. I realized I needed all the spiritual strength I could muster. I delved more deeply into Carol Ruth's lessons searching for tools to deal with this crisis. I also questioned why this would happen to Carol, who believed she was doing "God's work" as a psychotherapist. This naturally led me to ask, "Why was Carol Ruth, another woman doing 'God's work,' murdered?" From that came the question, "Where was God when Carol Ruth died?" "Where is God now that Carol has cancer?"

The book I had long planned took a dramatic turn: I would use Carol Ruth's lessons to try and cope with Carol's cancer as well as to seek God in Carol Ruth's murder and Carol's disease. This is the account of my search.

I am reluctant to mention the people who have made this book possible, only because the list is so long and I'm afraid I will inadvertently miss someone. First and foremost I want to thank the two Carols: Carol Ruth, my friend and spiritual mentor and Carol Martha, my love, best friend, muse, wife, and partner. I am blessed to have two such women in my life.

Two other women played a vital role in providing me with Carol Ruth's materials: Diana Gale did a remarkable job of gathering and preserving tapes of Sunday lessons; and Carlene Williams facilitated my acquiring these materials.

My thanks also go to Unity of Walnut Creek for granting permission to use Carol Ruth's writings and recordings. The librarians at Unity Village, Lee Summit, Missouri helped fill in some missing transcriptions. Shel and Jo Coudray graciously shared their memories of Carol Ruth in the years before I met her. Our friend, Kaye Thompson, introduced me to Adyashanti, whose teachings helped make the way clearer.

I deeply appreciate Greg Finch's non-judgmental

ear, which I have bent often with doubts and questions. Our Authentic Men's Community, especially Bob, Mark, Mark, Buck and Ron, have patiently listened and offered encouraging words as I have worked through my "stuff".

My friends, Reverend Beth Ann Suggs and Greg, read each chapter as I finished a draft and offered invaluable insights that helped make the final manuscript better. Another friend, Terry Docherty, read the final draft with the keen eye of the English teacher. My friend, Gail Derin, added her editorial skills to help create this finished book.

Our daughter, Elizabeth, helped me keep the writing "real" with her personal experience of the past year. The support of our children - Coy III, Elizabeth, Mellissa, and Susan and their families - has been beyond measure. Carol's mother, the Beautiful Kay, continues to inspire me and Carol's brother, Dave, is a source of quiet strength. The Prayer Chain of family and friends around the world constantly reminded Carol and me that we are loved and supported and never alone.

Lastly, I will never forget the Sutter Hospital staff, from administration to surgeons, who surrounded Carol with love while saving her life. I must mention especially our family doctor, Barbara Spinelli, the surgeons, Jay Owens and Michael Beneke, the oncologist, Stacy D'Andre, and the nurses and staff at the infusion center. These people are healing angels. Their compassion and professional skill exceeded all expectation. Our family and friends' prayers combined with Sutter's medical staff's ability have created miracles. For that, I am eternally grateful.

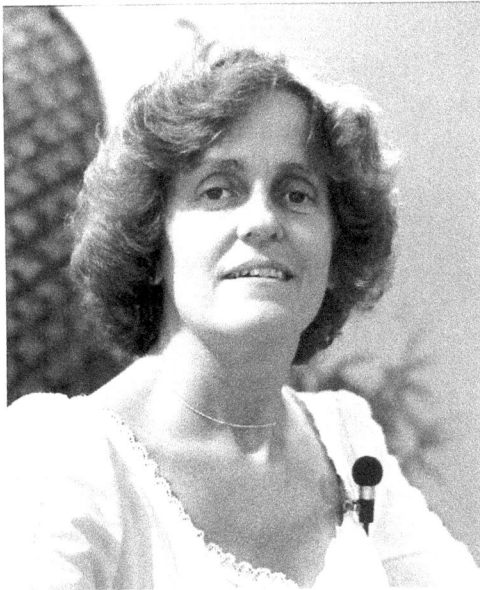

Carol Ruth Knox - 1984

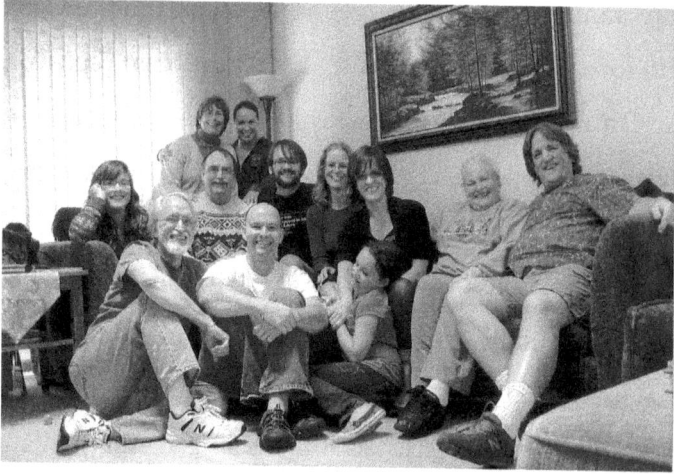

This is our family; they are very important to us. We didn't know how widely cancer affected people. Although Carol had the disease, every person in the family and friends had to deal with the disease.

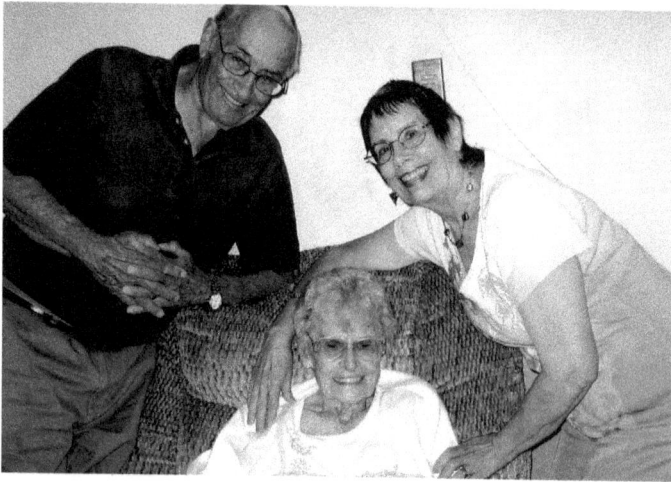

Brother Dave, Mother Kay, and Carol Martha - At times, contacting Kay was too painful for Carol. Her brother, Dave, stepped in and shouldered that load. Little acts of support like that can be priceless.

Introduction
by Carol Martha

Within these pages you will read of a man's journey, begun and ongoing in search of a relationship to God that would sustain him through all the challenges of his lifetime.

Coy and I met and married in midlife, having lived many chapters before "our chapter" began. I knew early in our courtship that he was a person of significance and my next stage was to be shared with him. I privately entertained the idea of being his "muse" as he contemplated writing a book on the teachings of Unity Minister Carol Ruth Knox, a book merging her teachings with his life events. How could her life's teachings guide him to absorb and accept her untimely, violent death? Could "God be in this, too"—as she always said?

Little did I know, years ago when I silently accepted the role of muse for Coy's book, that I would become the "life event" at the core of his work.

His evolving spiritual seeking had developed into daily practice wherein he created a loving, nurturing, safe, supportive environment for me to experience the full impact of my cancer, treatment and recovery. His being present and compassionate, yet holding a mature, safe container allowed me to decompensate, sink into unbridled anxiety, existential fears, and anger at God, and also allowed me to come out the other side into the joy of being alive, loved and accepted through it all. He helped me believe that all of it, the bitter and the sweet, was living non-duality.

As I have read his manuscript, I am inspired to use his teachings to find peace and understand God's intention as I begin this new chapter of my life.

May you, the reader, be touched by his offering and imagine "God is in this, too."

Carol Cross
Ovarian Cancer Survivor
November 2010

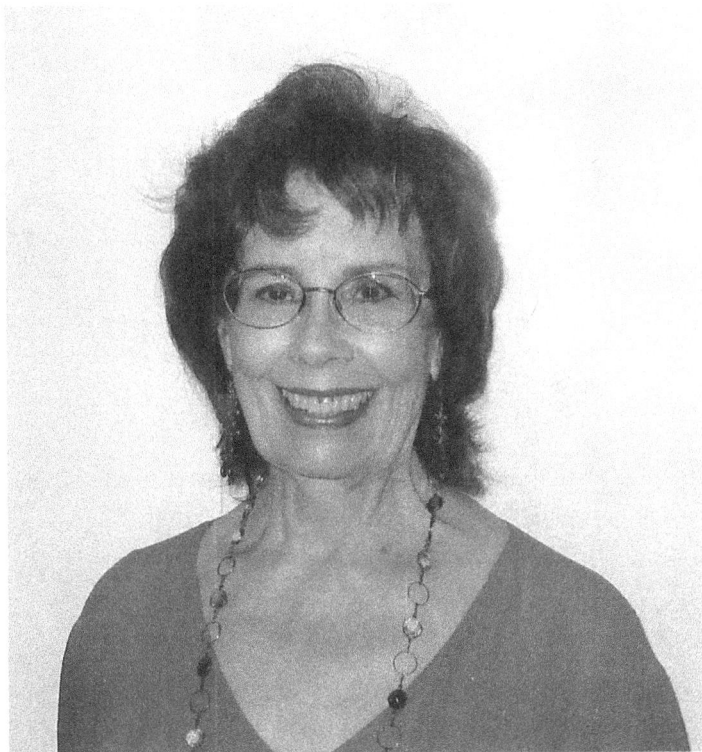

Carol Martha - 2010

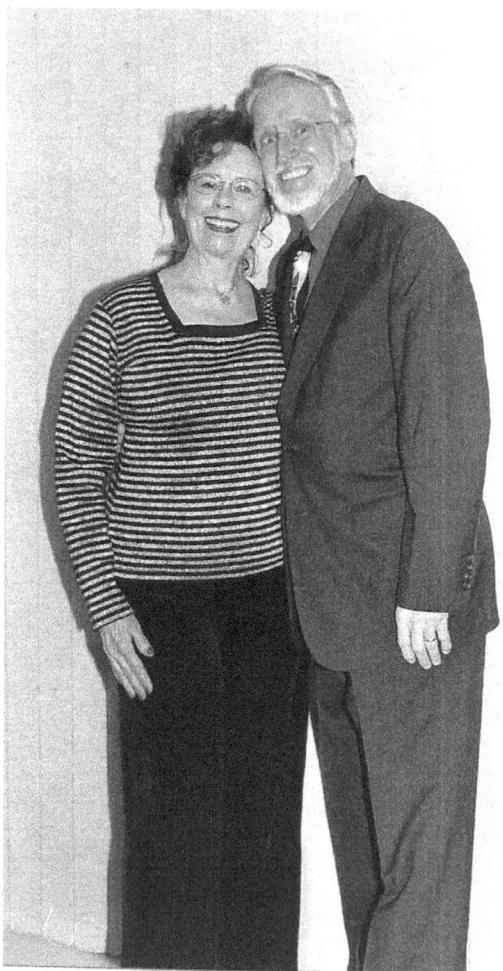

Carol Martha and Coy - 2008

Chapter 1 - This Can't Be Happening

Behind all this is a Divine knowing, which beholds that all levels are so, all is intended, nothing can be wrong, all is occurring at the same instant and nothing is more real or better than anything else.[i]

- Carol Ruth Knox

Life is our classroom. If we live consciously, life will present us the lessons we need for growth and we will see them as such.

- Coy Cross, The Author

May 28, 2009 is a sunny Thursday afternoon. My wife, Carol, and I sit holding hands without talking. We are waiting for her one o'clock appointment. Carol has not been feeling well, but has been too harried to really investigate the cause. Her 95-year-old mother, Kay, living in a care facility in Twin Falls, Idaho, 600 miles away, has suffered several serious health challenges this past year. Carol made six trips to Idaho in 2008 and two more trips earlier this year. A psychotherapist in private practice, Carol worries not only about her mother but that she has neglected her clients and her business during so much time away.

1

In fact, we have just returned from spending Mother's Day with Kay. Although abdominal pain caused Carol to consider delaying, she decided we would drive half way and then, if she felt well enough, continue on to Twin Falls. The importance of seeing her mother overshadowed the pain and we made the trip.

The day after reaching home on May 13, Carol saw our family doctor, Barbara Spinelli. Carol has a history of diverticulitis and we all believed it had reoccurred. Antibiotics did not relieve the symptoms, however, so Carol returned to Doctor Spinelli six days later. The doctor ordered lab tests, which revealed elevated cancer antigen-125 levels in Carol's blood stream. Doctor Spinelli then scheduled a CT scan for Friday, May 22. Memorial Day on Monday delayed the scan results until Tuesday, the 26th. That's the day Doctor Spinelli confirmed Carol had ovarian cancer. She referred Carol to Doctor Jay Owens, an oncology surgeon.

Carol asked Barbara, "If this were you, would Doctor Owens be the surgeon you trusted with your life?"

Barbara replied, "Absolutely! He is the best." She explained that after several years as a top surgeon in his field, he retired. Soon realizing he still had a passion for surgery and mentoring younger doctors, he resumed his practice.

On this sunny Thursday afternoon, Carol and I sit holding hands, without talking, waiting at the Roseville Sutter Medical Center to see him now.

Just the word "cancer" creates feelings of fear, hopelessness, and loss in me. I made the mistake of going on the internet and learning that only one of three women with ovarian cancer survives for five years.

Carol has been my best friend and partner in life for nearly twenty five years and my wife for twenty one. A really good person herself, she helps me be my "best self". She possesses an inner beauty that shines through to her entire persona. In addition to all that, we really like each other and cherish our time together. The thought of losing her seems unbearable. I can hardly look at her without tears filling my eyes.

Our friend Shirley, a registered nurse, arrives and we

introduce her as Carol's sister, so she can be with us during the appointment. She's here to provide moral support as well as a professional ear to hear subtleties we might miss.

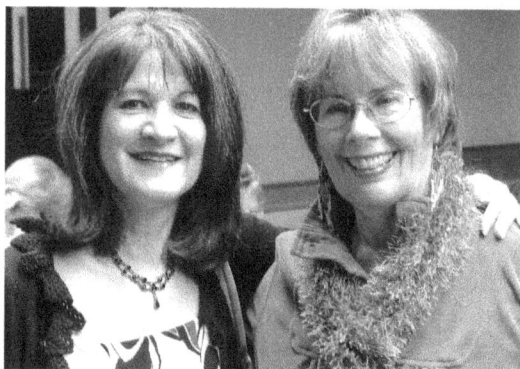

"Sister" Shirley and Carol (both moral support and professional)

Doctor Owens' nurse calls Carol's name and the three of us enter the examining room. Doctor Owens is a handsome, gray-haired man in his sixties. He quickly puts Carol and me at ease. Unlike other surgeons I have known, he seems kind and compassionate, not cold and aloof. He introduces his colleague, Michael Beneke, a younger surgeon who will assist in the surgery. I think to myself, "We get the best combination, years of experience and the latest medical training."

Showing us Carol's CT scan, Doctor Owens points

out where the cancer has already spread from her ovaries to other areas including the omentum, which is the tissue overlaying the stomach and intestines. This caused a fluid build-up in the abdomen and resulted in the recent weight gain that Carol couldn't "diet away". Based on the scan and her lab tests, he considers her cancer to be at Stage III, Level C. He adds that while ovarian cancer statistics can be alarming, each person is different. "You can be a success story and have a long and productive life. But, it is serious and we need to move quickly."

He explains the surgical procedure and reassures us that there is a good chance that surgery and chemotherapy will remove the cancer and destroy any remaining cells. During the surgery he will install two ports, one high on the chest and another at the bottom of the ribcage, for use during chemotherapy. When Carol expresses a reservation about the chemotherapy, Doctor Owens emphasizes, "For this to work, you need to be 'all in'!"

Carol agrees. "I'm all in," she says.

"It's a coincidence[1]," I think, "that Carol and I had talked just a few months before about what if one of us got cancer. We decided we would first rely on conventional medicine with an option for non-traditional therapy if the cancer recurred."

Doctor Owens tells us his nurse will call us with the time and date for the surgery. As Carol begins to cry softly, Owens puts his arm around her shoulder and says reassuringly, "We're going to take care of this."

Trying to absorb all we have been told, Shirley, Carol and I go to a nearby coffee shop to talk. Shirley answers questions we forgot to ask Owens and clarifies other questions where we are unsure.

A call awaits us at home: the first available operating room is Tuesday at Sutter General Hospital in Sacramento. Surgery is scheduled for one o'clock with an eleven a.m. check-in.

---

[1] I have come to believe there is no such thing as "coincidence". Everything is all part of a "Divine Plan".

We must immediately call and tell our children, who thankfully are all adults. We will go ahead with the already-planned birthday party for son Coy III and his wife Toni on Saturday. This will give us the opportunity to talk face-to-face with three of our children and their families. Sue, the youngest daughter, is temporarily working in New York and will be home next week.

Because Carol feels she cannot speak with her mother without crying, we call her brother Dave in Denver and ask him to break the news to Kay.

As we compile our to-do list, we keep repeating, "This doesn't seem real. I can't believe this is happening." But it is real and it is happening.

Carol spends Friday calling clients, many of whom have scheduled therapy appointments, explaining a medical emergency will prevent her from seeing them for several months. She gives each client three therapist names they can contact.

In another "coincidence", Carol had created a "professional will" a few days previously. Part of that included referral therapists who would see her clients immediately if anything happened to her. While closing her practice, even temporarily, is painful, her preplanning certainly makes the process more efficient.

While Carol is busy at her office, I meet my friend Greg. He is Shirley's husband. We meet at the nearby Peet's coffee shop.

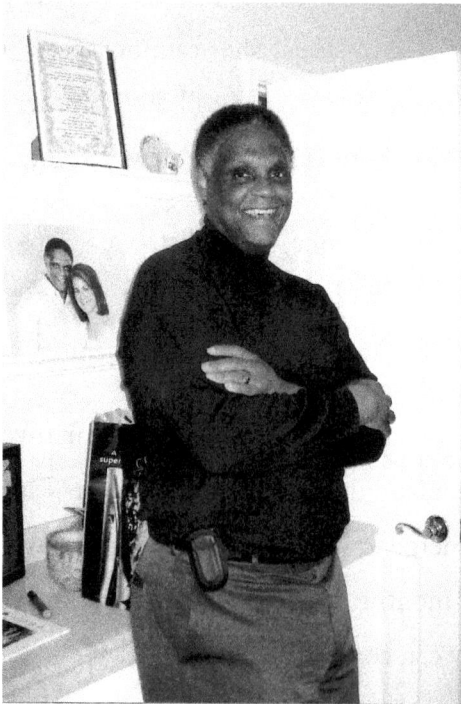

Greg - 2008

For the past twenty five years, Carol has been my confidante and the one with whom I could always share my deepest fears. But now I need someone, besides Carol or our immediate family, with whom I can express, not only my worries and my concerns about Carol's survival, but my doubts about my own ability to cope.

As Greg and I talk, I remind him that in 1982 my second wife Helen was seriously injured in an auto accident. Up to this point in my life I had learned to depend on myself and only on myself. "I can do this," I repeated it over and over even though I rationally knew it was impossible to do everything necessary to care for her, four children, my business and myself. Somehow I thought that "if I do all this and if I do it correctly and if I am very good, everything will be okay and Helen will get well. So, I didn't ask for help," I told Greg. "Instead, I dealt with the pain by numbing myself with alcohol. A year later, emotionally and physically exhausted, I considered suicide and only my love for my children and my elderly mother kept me from doing so. But I left the marriage and did not 'finish the job' of caring for Helen, our children, or myself."

Four years later, Jan, my first wife and the mother of

my three children, died in an auto accident. Four days later, my dad died from a stroke. Again, I "coped" with alcohol and "stuffed my feelings", becoming once more emotionally unavailable to support my children or others around me.

The two Carols, Carol Martha and Carol Ruth, helped me get through these dark days. I could rely on to them to help keep me anchored. When an intruder murdered my dear friend and mentor, Carol Ruth Knox, four months later, alcohol and stuffing my emotions was still my preferred method of dealing with life.

Yet, Carol Ruth's words kept coming into my awareness. I began studying her words and gradually understood more of what she had taught me. I started to see God's will in a new way. I realized I needed better coping mechanisms and to stop using alcohol as my crutch. But, I was not ready to directly confront the hurt and the loss.

In 2001 another car wreck killed my nineteen year-old grandson, Matt. It was devastating and although I chose not to numb myself with alcohol, I still "stuffed" my feelings and did not face the pain of his death and my daughter Elizabeth's agony.

Now I was facing Carol's traumatic disease. I knew I had to be different and I was afraid I would not be enough.

This time was different. The good news was, I finally figured out I didn't have to do this alone. I now have friends like Greg and the guys in our men's group, who will help me keep a better perspective. Our adult children are also available and very supportive. And, I know I can't heal Carol. Greg helps me understand my greatest gift to her is "to be consciously present."

I can "be." I now understand. I can consciously be myself and continue loving her.

I can consciously be present with and support her.

I can simply sit with her and consciously be present.

Leaving the coffee shop, I have more confidence about my role in supporting her and I realize, at the same time, I must release responsibility for the outcome. This dichotomy is absolutely critical. There are things that are in my control and things that are not. There are jobs that are mine to do, and aspects of this situation I can do nothing about. What I must focus on during this time of distress is being the best at what I can do and be.

No matter what I do, Carol could die. But how this "all turns out is none of my business." I must play *my part* to the best of my ability. I am well aware that this last twenty-four hours has already changed my life dramatically and permanently.

As I reach Carol's office, I pause outside and talk to God for a moment. "Okay, there is a pattern here. Obviously, you have an important spiritual lesson for me. This time I promise to stay conscious and open and learn what you are teaching. I don't want to have to take this class again."

At the same time, I am aware of the magnitude of the blessing that this experience offers. This is a moment of great insight for me. Although I feel great pain at the very real possibility of losing the woman I deeply love, I also see the higher level opportunity for spiritual growth this presents for both Carol and me.

As I open the door to Carol's office, I begin the job

that is mine to do. I help Carol. I help our family and friends deal with her cancer. This time I am determined to do it consciously.

Saturday is a day of joy and laughter tempered by worry and fear with some crying mixed in as we celebrate the two birthdays with our children and grandchildren. We are all aware that it will be a while before we can be together like this again. Carol and I reassure our family that she has great doctors and the surgery and chemotherapy will kill all the cancer and she will have a long, happy life. Our family probably realizes we are trying to convince ourselves as well as them.

Sunday, Carol and I drive over to Stinson Beach, our favorite "getaway" just north of San Francisco. The ocean is where we both can feel God's presence. We walk down the beach to "our" private spot and spread beach towels, and sit a while. As the sun rises in the sky, we lie back and listen to the waves wash against the shore and the occasional call of the seagulls. I am consciously present here with her.

There are few words between us, but this is a special

shared moment. We both feel our great love for each other, so words seem unnecessary. After a late lunch, we drive home, again with little talk, both lost in our own thoughts.

Monday is surgery prep day, which means preparing both physically and mentally. Although each of us fears surgery will reveal the cancer has spread beyond the point where medical treatment can kill it, we don't voice that. Our talk is filled with last minute tasks yet to be done and names of people we still need to contact. Finally, we agree that any more notification will have to be by e-mail, repeating the news via telephone has become too difficult. I create an e-mail list of family and friends whom I can ask for love, support and prayers. In return, I promise to keep them updated on Carol's condition.

Right in the middle of compiling our list, a neighbor with a dead car battery asks for a ride to the auto parts store. Not knowing of Carol's diagnosis, he casually asks how I'm doing.

"I feel like I was just kicked in the testicles so hard I

can hardly catch my breath," I reply. At his shocked expression, I explain what's happening.

The rest of the day is mostly quiet, interrupted occasionally by Carol's reminders of "be sure and remember to..." pay some bill or send a friend's birthday card, things she normally does, but for which I now will be responsible.

Underneath the busyness of detailing future chores, Carol must be thinking because on Monday evening she announces, "Tomorrow, when I go to the hospital, I am going to tell everyone I come in contact with, 'All the hands that touch me are the hands of God!' "

This is the prayer and affirmation our friend Linda shared with us years ago before her successful surgery. Carol has often passed this prayer onto her clients when any of them faced illness. Now, she will seek comfort in it herself.

As I ponder the spiritual lessons contained in all this pain, I wish I could talk with my friend Carol Ruth Knox, the dynamic minister of Unity Center, Walnut Creek, who had played an important role in both my wife Carol's and my lives. I first met Carol Ruth in 1980 when she spoke at the small Unity Church in Modesto, California. She and I both felt an instant "connection." A few months later I moved to Walnut Creek and we quickly became friends.

She was a charismatic speaker who had the ability to explain complex ideas so that everyone in the audience could understand. Also, Carol Ruth experienced God in everyday life and brought that to her Sunday talks. Her Sunday sermons became so popular, the Center had to expand to three services and Easter Sunday services filled a local theater. Her classes included lessons from all the world religions, because she knew God spoke in every language and to all people.

It took me five years of searching for "what is missing in my life" before I found this mentor. She helped me see a God *always* present in the *entire* Universe, a God as the *only* power, and a God that *knows everything*: omnipresence, omnipotence and omniscience. I took several classes with her and served on her church's board of directors until I returned to school in Santa Barbara. Carol Ruth and I loved each other as dear friends.

She helped me through several personal crises, including when my second wife Helen suffered a serious head injury in a traffic accident. Carol Ruth remained my friend a couple of years later when I realized I had to leave that marriage. She had been there to lean on when my first wife Jan, the mother of my three children, and my dad both died within the same week. She could always help me see from a larger perspective and helped me eventually come to realize that "God was in this, too." Carol Ruth often described life as a dance with the Divine (her Boston accent pronounced it "dhance with the Divine"), but right now I don't feel like dhancing. Carol Ruth is dead, murdered by an intruder and it feels like my dhance partner is stepping all over my feet.

Suddenly, I realize that although Carol Ruth is dead, I can still turn to her for help. When she died I had been too caught up in the circumstances surrounding her death and engrossed in the pain to look for God. But her lessons are still available to help me deal with this painful time. "Coincidentally," again, I recently began writing a book on the life-lessons I learned from her. In preparation, I accumulated hundreds of her Sunday lessons and copies of almost everything she wrote and have spent the last two years listening to her talks and reading her messages. I believe her words will give me the strength I will need to confront Carol's cancer. I will "practice what Carol Ruth preached" and see if it works or, perhaps, I'll discover the beliefs that I hold most dear have no application in life and are mere metaphysical bullshit.

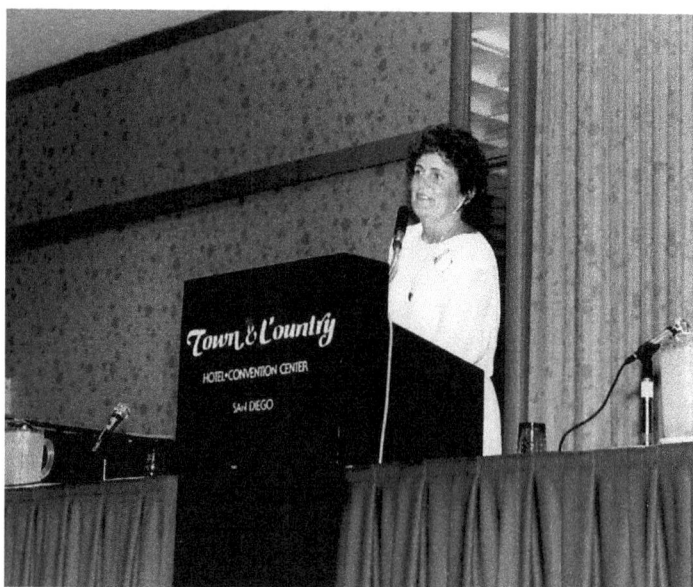

Carol Ruth Knox at Unity Minister's Conference - 1986

Chapter 2 - A Unity Minister

[L]ife is not always fair; it does not always add up, figure out or work as we would have it, nor does it make sense or justify. The step into the third dimension is to understand that there is some deeper intention, and that deeper intention cannot always be seen. Thus it forces us to give up and to step deeper within, deeper. When one touches that dimension, one touches the spiritual and gets behind the brain.[ii]

- Carol Ruth Knox

Life has kicked me in the testicles enough times that I now release my filters and stop trying to keep certain experiences away. I let my entire life in. As if I had another choice!

- Coy Cross, The Author

Carol's diagnosis immediately returns me to 1982. It's Friday, December 10th. Helen and I have been married for fourteen months and are very much in love. We moved to Walnut Creek from Modesto last year and bought a house cleaning service with about a dozen employees. Helen left early this morning for a final property settlement hearing with her first husband in Modesto. When the phone rings a little after ten a.m., I think it is an employee with a problem. Instead, it's the California Highway Patrol, "There's been an accident.

Helen's in the Livermore General Hospital. They need your signature for surgery." When I arrive at the hospital I learn a large cement truck had broadsided Helen's small Triumph Spitfire and she has suffered a major injury to her brain's left side.

Thus began my previous great spiritual lesson, but one about which I am still realizing new dimensions. I had been studying with Carol Ruth Knox for about eighteen months and I immediately begin applying her teachings as I understood them. I first pray Helen will survive until I reach the hospital, and she does. I now pray she will live through surgery, and she does. She spends the next two weeks in a coma. I pray she will awaken from the coma, and she does. Over the next four months I pray she will recognize me, talk, walk, and she does. Then I pray she will completely recover and return to the Helen I fell in love with, but she doesn't. What happened? I practice every spiritual principle I know and nothing works. Seeing no results, I gradually slide into deep depression.

Carol Ruth had spoken of the "Dark Night of the Soul," but I believed that was reserved for saints or at least beings more spiritually evolved than I. I did not consider myself spiritually aware enough to be worthy of a "Dark Night" experience; God must have been punishing me for leaving my previous marriage. I now realize my short time with Carol Ruth provided me with only a beginner's understanding of her teachings. From today's perspective I can readily see I had expected God to intercede and produce my specific desired outcome. Since God apparently had acceded to my preliminary requests, I didn't understand when He/She/It did not grant the big one. I expected God to let me be in charge of how it all turned out. How egotistical is that?

Even though I continue to learn from 1982, I can't linger there. I must be present in the present. As I begin my search into Carol Ruth's Sunday lessons and other materials for tools to deal with Carol's cancer, I acknowledge my approach will take time. I know the answers will not be found through my intellect. But if I let myself feel the depths of my sadness and my fear, I'm afraid visions of a dark life without Carol will overwhelm me. If that happens, I cannot be here, consciously present with and for her. Being consciously present with her and for her is what I can and must do.

So I fall back on what I know and what I tend to revert to first, my intellect and my training as a professional historian. I will carefully read and study Carol Ruth's materials looking for answers, answers that my deeper awareness understands lie within me. This intellectual approach will keep my mind busy and away from my darker thoughts until I can gradually open to my deeper feelings and intuitive nature where my real answers are.

Turning to Carol Ruth's Sunday lesson quoted above, she says there is a Divine intent behind the events of our life and "nothing can be wrong" and "nothing is more real or better than anything else." If I am to confront Carol's cancer consciously, I must be able to see "God is in this, too" and "there is some deeper intention." I have always relied on my intellect for solutions, but I know I must eventually seek answers "behind the brain" in the spiritual. I believe Carol Ruth will help me find my own path "to step deeper within."

When I met Carol Ruth in 1980, she had already served as Walnut Creek Unity Center's minister for ten years and had "grown up in Unity." I, on the other hand, had only recently discovered New Thought and learned metaphysics could be something other than a branch of philosophy.

As a child in Southeastern Kentucky, Baptist and Adventist Christian churches shaped my vision of God, prayer, the world and my place in it.

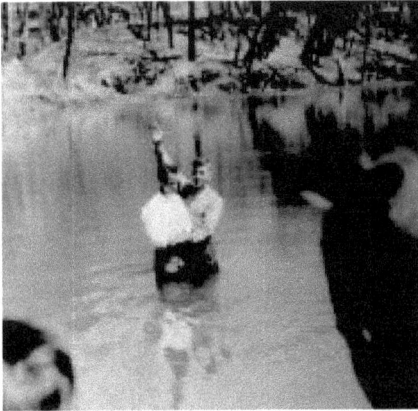

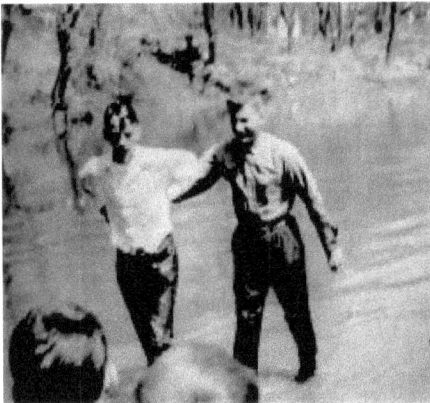

Coy baptized at age fourteen

I later became a teenaged-thorn in the ministers' and elders' sides constantly questioning church teachings. "Why is the punishment for minor offenses and horrendous crimes the same: eternal damnation in a fiery hell?" "How can God trust Satan to keep sinners in hell? It seems to me that Satan would want to reward sinners and, therefore, could not be trusted to punish them. I think he would allow them to run free, especially the most evil and despicable ones." "Why did God create Satan in the first place?" "Why does God let horrible things happen to innocent children?" "Why is watching a movie in a theater a sin, while watching the same movie at home on television is not?" "How can I live my daily life and avoid 'worldly things'? Exactly what are 'worldly things' anyway?" Because I could never find adequate answers and feeling a deep sense of guilt from my constant misdeeds or impure thoughts, even though I was a good kid, I left the church as a teenager. By my twenties, I had become an obnoxious agnostic, asking the same questions of anyone who dared express their faith around me.

Years later, I began to doubt my doubt when a class in the anatomy and physiology of the human eye convinced me that this body is too marvelous to have evolved by chance. This realization coupled with an uneasy feeling that grew into unrest and then emptiness convinced me something was missing from my life. There had to be more to life than what I was experiencing. That's when I began my quest for "something more". I first looked in familiar churches, but my answers were not there. After a couple of years, I found a non-denominational church with a charismatic minister and a dynamic congregation. I thought I was 'home'. A few weeks later, however, the minister's Sunday sermon seemed to say, "No matter what we do, everything is going to get worse and worse."

I thought I must have misheard, so I asked a church elder and he confirmed that I had heard correctly. Still the questioner, I proposed, "Say, for example, I am the most gifted evangelist ever born and I convert every living person on the planet to Christianity, will things still get worse and worse?" When he replied "Yes," I said, "I'm sorry. I don't believe that."

I shared my story and my frustration with a friend, who suggested Unity. Having never heard of Unity, I asked, "What's that?" After his brief description, I had doubts, but agreed to check it out. My first exposure to "affirmations and denials" sounded to me like a positive thinking sales pitch, but at least the minister wasn't saying "things are going to get worse and worse." The teaching seemed so foreign to me I wanted to learn its foundation and the church's background. The need to first satisfy my intellect led me to begin studying church history and the writings of the co-founders Charles and Myrtle Fillmore.

Unity itself evolved in the late nineteenth century from the Transcendentalist and New Thought movements. Finding no conventional cure for her tuberculosis, Myrtle Fillmore and husband Charles attended a class on spiritual health where she learned a new way to pray. Instead of pleading with God for healing, she affirmed, "I am a child of God, and therefore I do not inherit sickness."[iii] Within two years she experienced a complete healing.

Charles, although lacking much formal education, had an inquisitive mind and sought a scientific explanation for Myrtle's cure. He concluded God is not an external, personal, arbitrary monarch who rules the Universe as I had been taught, but spirit that dwells within each of us. God, therefore, is immanent and transcendent, both within us "nearer than our hands and feet" and everywhere present, even the far reaches of the Universe.

Charles Fillmore was a believer in both science and metaphysics[2]. He saw the Bible as an allegory for the evolving human consciousness, with innumerable examples of mental and spiritual laws. Spiritual laws could not be confirmed through physical experiments, which relied on the five senses. But Fillmore believed that knowledge gained through intuition and prayer was as valid as information acquired through the senses; therefore, spiritual laws could be "scientifically" proven and duplicated through repeated demonstrations and

---

[2] Metaphysics: "The systematic study of the science of Being; that which transcends the physical. By pure metaphysics is meant a clear understanding of the realm of ideas and their legitimate expression." Charles Fillmore, *The Revealing Word*, (Unity Village MO: Unity Books, 1959).

personal experiences. Fillmore called this approach "practical Christianity" since we can improve our health, prosperity or happiness by applying these metaphysical and divine truths to our daily life. Prayer is the path to alignment with God. "The purpose of prayer," according to Charles Fillmore, "is to change your thinking. God does not change." [iv]

This answers one of the questions I kept asking as a kid, "Why does God answer sometimes and not others?"

Unlike other religions, Unity has "no dogmas or creeds" and does not rely on revelation for its authority. Fillmore added that Unity students are not to believe anything which they cannot logically demonstrate to be true. Unity ministers, including Carol Ruth Knox, therefore, base their teachings not only on principles developed in Fillmore's writings, but also on other spiritual traditions and each minister's own divine insights. Each Unity center is unique and reflects its minister's spiritual development and interests.

I appreciate the solid philosophical and scientific foundation Charles Fillmore gave the Unity movement.

Although Fillmore satisfies my intellect, I can't "think my way to God." I agree with his statement that I can find God through my mind, but my path to God is through intuition and not intellect. I believe God must be experienced. So I accept Fillmore's teachings, but continue seeking my own answers. I must remember to keep telling myself, "Stay out of your head, move into the heart where the answers are found!" Carol Ruth continues to speak to both my head and my heart.

She notes the Fillmores considered themselves teachers, not ministers. As a spiritual leader, her highest goal was not to "minister to" people, but to give them principles to use in their daily lives. Even now I recall attending every Sunday service she gave from September 1984 through June 1985 and each Sunday leaving with a new insight or realization of God active in my daily life.

By summer 1985, Helen and I had been separated for more than two years and I was slowly recovering from my darkest period following her accident. I even started pondering what I wanted to do with the rest of my life. I finally decided to pursue my long-held dream of a doctorate degree in history. I applied and was accepted at the University of California, Santa Barbara. For the first time, I would be able to concentrate on school full-time without a job or family to consider. I was responsible for no one but myself. I was starting a new life and I was excited.

As a Walnut Creek Unity board member who lived near the church, I stopped by several times a week to sign checks. While there I couldn't help notice an attractive volunteer who often worked in the office. I had met Carol Martha a few years earlier, while we were both married, but I didn't really know her. In July 1985, we were both single, but I was leaving soon and had no room in my new life for a relationship. Still, I was drawn to her. I finally asked her to lunch and she accepted. After lunch, she gave me the most delicious hug I had ever received. Even though my head said "not now," my heart knew I wanted to see her again. We were soon spending almost every day together, each aware that my move to Santa Barbara (a six hour car ride) was rapidly approaching.

Two weeks before my classes started, my daughter Beth called saying she had left her husband and needed to see me. While talking with her I realized she was experiencing some psychological problem that was far beyond my capability. I called my new friend Carol Martha, who was studying to be a marriage and family therapist, and explained what was happening. She suggested I bring Beth to see her. She recognized that Beth needed hospitalization to treat what was later diagnosed as bi-polar disorder. Carol and I took Beth to the local mental health facility, where she was admitted. Throughout the crisis, Carol proved herself a great friend whom I could count on for support. She was my partner when I needed a partner most. I knew then this was a quality person who possessed all the attributes I admired and desired in a woman. She was smart, fun to be with, spiritually inquisitive, the most honest person I had ever met, and a true friend. Plus, she was beautiful and extremely sexy. But, we were both adamant that we would never marry again. So we decided to just let our relationship unfold.

In September 1985, I moved to Santa Barbara and returned to school. Carol stayed in the Bay Area while finishing her senior year at San Francisco State. Yet, we spent most weekends together, either I drove up or she drove down. I put a lot of miles on a 1963 Volkswagen Bug that year. After she completed her bachelor's degree, she applied to U.C. Santa Barbara and was accepted into the counseling psychology program. In 1986 we moved in together, but were still determined we would not marry again. Later that year my first wife Jan died in an auto accident and five days later my dad died. Carol again loved and supported me and my children. Three months later, Carol Ruth Knox was killed and Carol was by my side as I grieved the triple loss. By Christmas 1987, I knew I wanted this woman with me forever and asked her to marry me. She agreed and we married on Valentine's Day 1988.

Now as I face the possibility of losing my wife, my friend, my partner and my forever love, I turn to my other friend Carol for answers. As I read Carol Ruth's small book on Unity, she explains, "Unity is a blending of the Eastern and Western traditions." She, therefore, considers herself to be a "Universalist," believing all major religions contain Truth[3] and ultimately lead to God. I believe this, too. "The core of Unity teachings is mystical…When you are looking for answers through the Unity process, Unity will say, 'Go within.'"[v] Carol Ruth calls those who attended her classes or church services Truth students, of whom she says, "The first significant statement given to any student of Truth is to tell them that we cannot tell anybody what God is; therefore you are required to search for yourself. Most of all, search to experience It for yourself. We suggest that you do the searching inside, and the silence is the proper place in which to do that searching"[vi] I was and still am one of her Truth students and this directs me back to meditation. Some of my deepest insights have come while sitting in "the silence".

In Christian teachings, God is the first of the Holy

---

[3] Truth with a capital "T" indicates a divine or universal truth that never changes, i.e., "I am a child of God." Truth with a small "t" reflects a statement that may be true today, but could change later, i.e., "My car is new."

Trinity. The second is Jesus. Unity differentiates between "Jesus" and "the Christ[4]." "Jesus" is the man, the human incarnation. "The Christ" is God's perfect expression within each of us. Carol Ruth explains that I was born with this indwelling Christ and I looked at the world without judgments. When I was hungry, I cried. If I was content, I smiled. I judged neither as better than the other. At that stage, I was expressing my true essence. Quickly I developed thinking and feeling systems and learned to consider pleasant experiences good and unpleasant ones bad. I soon came to believe that my true self was the body that felt the pain or pleasure and forgot that I was really "the indwelling Christ."[vii]

Carol Ruth calls the Holy Spirit, the final part of the Holy Trinity, the "catalytic agent" or "connecting force"

---

[4] Jesus-"The Man of Nazareth, son of Mary; the Savior of mankind according to present-day Christian belief." Christ-"The incarnating principle of the God-man; the perfect Word or idea of God." Fillmore, *The Revealing Word.*

that pushes me toward God. Her role, as she defines it, is to trigger a hunger, "maybe even through anger and outrage," that her students would release and allow "the flame of Spirit to become active." In describing the experience, she says, "Much of the pain is caused by this pressure pushing on you to become vulnerable, open, awakened and available to a larger dimension of yourself." If I am willing to accept the pain as growth and to "live at the full edge of [my] potential, then [I am] being born continually breaking the shells of encrustations over and over again so that [I] might come out, through one more egg, one more crust, one more crack, one more edge, into a new world."[viii]

Wow! Twenty-five years ago, she perfectly described my pain, my anger, my hunger that is forcing me into this inner journey to find God in Carol Martha's cancer. I am willing to become "vulnerable, open, awakened and available to a larger dimension of" myself. I know this search will leave me forever changed and living in "a new world".

Carol Ruth cautions that recognizing I am one with God will not necessarily make me healthier or wealthier.

"It is like a light, a sun, a force, that is indomitable in the face of anything external. Remember, that having such a force does not mean that the external is easy; you still can lose your homes, relationships, money, life [can] still [be] hard [or] easy."[ix] But, she promises, I "will experience more of a sense of the Presence, a feeling of security, an absence of fear, a freedom and a conviction while living…[I] may not show any worldly results because that is not what this power is about. It is about connection and inner power and freedom from fear."[x] My hope is that connecting with God will allow me to consciously "be" with Carol Martha as she confronts her surgery and the chemotherapy that comes after.

Carol Ruth abhorred the superficial and platitudes and admitted she often felt like "an outcast," an outcast who denied the existence of sin, which other Unity minister often called "missing the mark." "Missing the mark just throws you into duality" and implies that you are then separate from God. "I don't teach either/or, I teach both and I don't teach any kind of rejection of anything… it is all total acceptance…there is no way for there to be separation [from God]."[xi][5] Life, for her, had become a prayer, a prayer that maintained her in "constant grace." In grace she knew "that nothing could be out of order" and that it was "all perfect" just as it was.[xii] Were Carol Ruth's murder and my Carol's cancer "all perfect"? Carol Ruth would say they were. That is the place I want to get to and I believe she can still teach me how, even now, more than twenty years after her death.

Carol Ruth describes a person's growth and development along a spiritual path as "the soul's evolution" and created a chart outlining the process *(see Process Chart Appendix A)*. Many people are born and spend their entire lifetime at an "unconscious" level, with little or no ego. They consider themselves "victims"

---

[5] This is "non-duality," the belief that God is the only presence, the only power and the only knowledge in the Universe and in our lives. Therefore, there is no right or wrong, good or bad, light or dark. We are all one with everything and everything is God unfolding.

with no control over their life. She notes they are living at an instinctual level. "A large amount of their nature and behavior is functioning from the instinctual carryover of genes and heritage. . . . No one ever totally gives up 'Victim'; sometimes we can even learn to play 'Victim' and do it well. . . . The energy and desire barely exist. In fact, you don't even care. . . . [S]ome people never leave childhood consciousness, Victim." [xiii]

My own experience growing up in Kentucky in a fundamentalist church coincides with this Victim consciousness. I considered myself an "evil sinner," who could never be otherwise. I tried to avoid "worldly" activities, although I could not get a clear distinction of what was worldly and what was not. I spent most of my time feeling guilty and confused. I knew I could never be as perfect as Jesus, so I was already doomed to hell. If I was headed for hell within the church, then why continue trying? I might as well leave the church and enjoy some of the "worldly things".

Sometimes a "Victim" sees a television show, reads a book or hears an upbeat Sunday sermon that causes them to question previously held beliefs. Something awakens a seed of belief "I can have some control over my life. It doesn't always have to be this way...I want control. I want power. I want to have an effect. I want to create a reality. I want to stand up and be counted...I want to go beyond my limits as a Victim."[xiv] Positive thinking books and seminars, affirmations and denials, and New Thought churches, such as Unity, can stimulate and reinforce ego growth until the person moves out of Victim-hood. My own transition started when I became fed-up with feeling guilty all the time.

Unity teaches we are God's children and, as such, we are not horrible sinners, but beloved offspring. God is not the jealous, vengeful, capricious being located in some distant heaven portrayed in my earlier "Victim" training, but a loving presence within each of us. This helped me see myself as a child of a loving God, not the perpetual sinner who constantly offended a vengeful God. Furthermore, consciously working with God, we can co-create the life we want. Unity's Sunday services stress our infinite potential and evening classes on prosperity and positive thinking explain the steps. At this level the person uses "visioning" and "treasure mapping" to manifest jobs, automobiles, houses or relationships to fulfill their goals and desires. We can become "Victor" over our life situations.[xv]

Some "Victors," who apparently have everything a person could want, however, become discontented and realize that possessions and "externals" no longer satisfy. "The exciting internal nature of this process is that the effect has its limits...You find out that it is possible to move into another realm of expression as you observe people and life itself has something else to offer." Carol Ruth calls this new realm "Vehicle," but the movement from "Victor" to "Vehicle" includes passing through "The Dark Night of the Soul," the experience Saint John of the Cross detailed in a book by the same name. In describing her own "Dark Night," she writes of a "life-hurt that brought forth anguish, despair, a feeling of loss and loneliness" deeper than any she had ever felt before. Although most people resist "The Dark Night," Carol Ruth strongly urges "one must allow oneself to go into it...The main message as one goes through is to realize it is all right...This process, this feeling, is right."[xvi]

I have wondered about the "Dark Night" experience

for nearly thirty years. In 1983, following Helen's accident, I withdrew into myself, became depressed, considered suicide. Two years later we divorced. Although it felt like my survival was at stake, I have felt guilty for "failing" to live up to my standards of how a man "should be." Recently, a series of seemingly unrelated events has given me new insight into that period. A few weeks ago, as part of a six-month training to become a more authentic man, I created a rite of passage for other men in the program. In the ritual, we formed a circle and each man in turn knelt and was baptized with water and the words, "I bless you and see you as an authentic man. I wash away the ordinary man and welcome this authentic man into our circle of authentic men."

A week later, at a men's workshop, the facilitator spilled a jar of stones in the center of our circle and each man selected one that appealed to him. Then we envisioned our stone's "life cycle" from its creation to the present. Sharing afterwards, we replaced the rock in the story with ourselves and recounted the story as our autobiography. My rock moved from a quiet beach down to the depths of the ocean to be reborn and carried by the tides back to the beach.

The third, seemingly unconnected, occurrence came a few days later when a letter from my ex-wife Helen arrived. Her letters normally produce a flood of guilt. But, suddenly, I could see my 1982-83 experiences with new eyes. I know her accident and the aftermath changed me. I became aware that "I am not in charge. There is a force much larger than I controlling the world. My challenge is to be in sync with that force." Now I realize the period after her accident was my baptism, my "Dark Night," but instead of accepting it and flowing with it, I tried to bury it under a sea of guilt and alcohol. By resisting the painful entry into the "Dark Night," I extended the period of suffering for years. With this new awareness, twenty-five years of guilt seems to have lifted. Time will show if this is permanent. My friend, Reverend Beth Ann Suggs, pointed out, "Your experience with Carol's cancer is another Dark Night of the Soul!" I replied, "It doesn't feel the same. I am not experiencing the depth of despair that I went through before." Her response, "That's because you have been growing and learning. Write about how you are doing that." Carol's cancer has given me a "do-over" and the chance to "get it right" this time.

Carol Ruth explains the "Dark Night" is necessary preparation for the "Vehicle" level or one she also calls "consciously not conscious." In this new state of "beingness", the ego and personality are still present, but diminished and softened. There is a desire for quiet and stillness. I can gain understanding, clarity and a greater appreciation for all life. I will trade my personal will for Divine will. An awareness of "being lived through" then arises. This is the stage of "acceptance of what is," this is the place where I can see God in everything, including Carol's cancer.[xvii] I have long believed that Jesus brought a positive message of love, brotherhood and forgiveness, but the churches I grew up with and many others preached that only a "chosen few" were acceptable to God. Now I know we are all not only "acceptable" but "beloved" of God.

But "the soul's evolution" is not a straight line. Carol Ruth, when using the Victim-Victor-Vehicle model to illustrate her point, always drew a large infinity sign that stretched from Vehicle to Victim. She says we do not reach Vehicle and stay there. Life's events create a constant flow that can cause us to drop from functioning at the Vehicle level to the Victim level almost instantly.[6]

This movement from "Victor" to "Victim" coincides with my own early experience in Unity. Shortly after discovering Unity, I became a member of the church and served on the board of directors. I attended classes and joined a Mastermind group determined to create my own business. Two years later, I owned a business, which "proved" to me that I was a "Victor." A few months later a large truck struck Helen's small car and she suffered traumatic head injuries. I quickly slipped back into "Victim-hood". A year later I was so depressed and in such emotional distress I seriously considered ending my life. Even "Victors" cannot always remember to co-create everything. With Carol Ruth's death I

---

[6] Don Richard Riso and Russ Hudson give an even more detailed explanation of these "Levels of Development" in their book, *The Wisdom of the Enneagram: The Complete Guide to Psychological and Spiritual Growth for the Nine Personality Types* (New York: Bantam Books, 1999), 75-94

again immediately returned to the "Victim" place, I had lost someone precious in my life. But, more and more I am able to see her death as a turning point in my soul's growth. I am now confronting an even greater milestone with Carol's cancer.

In *Unity: A Spiritual Path*, Carol Ruth suggests a spiritual practice for connecting to God. She cautions the seeker must totally let go of control, while at the same time realizing "You are a grand experiment. You are part of the experiment because God's experiment with Himself becoming you" is not complete yet. She cites an Albert Einstein quote, "God is a scientist, not a magician," to illustrate her point, then concludes, "This is a wonderful opportunity for you to explore, for you to ignite yourself, for you to discover what you are about."[xviii]

The simple, but not easy, spiritual practice she recommends is first, "You must carry a prayer in your heart." Second, "You must meditate daily." Third, "Clean up your body." And, fourth, "Practice and exercise discipline." In summary, "Practice the prayer ongoing, full-time. Do the spadework of meditation.

Clean up your body and exercise, bringing the whole system together...Practice and discipline. And then, consent... to the way God is operating life in your system. Do not ignore any part of your life or call it by any name except God."[xix]

Reading her words, listening to her voice and seeing her face in the videos brings me both joy and pain: the joy of seeing once again how wonderful she was and still is, and the pain of realizing how much I still miss physically talking and being with her. Sometimes I find myself becoming so absorbed in a video, that I forget for a brief moment that she is dead; then suddenly I am flooded with sadness when I return to the present. But now, at least, I have a place to start. I see the journey to my "deeper within" as parallel paths of studying Carol Ruth's lessons and committing to the practices she recommends.

But I know now that neither Carol Ruth, nor the Fillmores, nor the Bible, nor the Bhagavad-Gita, nor St. John of the Cross, nor the hundreds of other spiritual teachers whose books I have read have my answers. If wisdom came from book knowledge, I should be able to walk on water by now. Spiritual leaders can only provide the tools and point to a direction for us to consider. What I seek can only come through my own intuition and insight from my personal connection with God. I will begin with prayer.

Chapter 3 - Prayer

And Ruth said . . . whither thou goest, I will go; and where thou lodgest, I will lodge . . .

- Ruth 1:16

The word "prayer" has no absolute meaning in our day. It means one thing to the child who says, "Now I lay me down to sleep." It means something entirely different to the person who says his "Our Fathers" unthinkingly in a monotonous drone. It means one thing to the person who sits quietly under the trees in a wordless adoration of life and nature and with a receptivity to the "still small voice" of Spirit. It means another thing to the congregation of the preacher who gives a twenty-minute prayer that is eloquent and studied, and that touches every area of human need.[xx]

- Eric Butterworth, Unity minister

Our tendency has been, in our growing up with prayer, to think that we are that little boy who keeps ordering God what to do, thereby putting God outside and thinking that somehow we can bring God down to our level.[xxi]

- Carol Ruth Knox

I don't sleep much between Thursday's appointment with the surgeons and Tuesday's surgery date. When I'm not reassuring Carol and our family or notifying friends, I'm reminiscing about our nearly twenty-five years together or recalling everything I've ever known, heard, or experienced about prayer. Carol agreed to marry me while I was a graduate student with dubious job prospects. The morning after I submitted my dissertation, I received a phone call offering me a job as an Air Force historian. I quickly accepted, but the position was at Scott Air Force Base in southern Illinois and I was to begin work in three weeks. Without hesitation, Carol readily agreed, we would load our possessions onto a Ryder truck and move to Illinois, even though she knew the move meant interrupting her own career-path to becoming a marriage and family therapist. Harder yet for both of us, we would be two thousand miles away from our children and grandchildren. Years later, she recounted sitting in Carol Ruth's Prayer of the Heart weekend workshop at Unity the month after we started dating. In her heart she carried the question, "What am I to do with this man?" The answer came, "Be as Ruth." Pondering this response, she remembered Ruth's promise to her mother-in-law Naomi, "Whither thou goest, I will go." For the past twenty-five years, this is what she has done. This is the wife and partner I now might lose. This is too painful to think about, so I try to pray.

Not long ago, if you had asked me, "Do you know how to pray?" I would have considered the question ludicrous. "Of course I know how to pray. I have been praying since I was a small child." Then, in anticipation of writing a book based on Carol Ruth's teachings, I took a serious and objective look at prayer. My thoughts and beliefs on prayer become more important and more immediate as my wife Carol and I prepare for her surgery. To inform our extended biological and spiritual family of Carol's diagnosis and keep them aware of her progress, we create an e-mail list that includes people of many faiths and living around the world. My request is "Keep us in your thoughts and prayers." It does not matter to me how people pray or to whom they direct their prayers, I want their consciousness united in supporting the best outcome for Carol. Now, I have to confess, I feel like a hypocrite. Not only do I not know how to pray, but I am not even sure what prayer is. When my need seems the greatest, I am more unsure than ever. If God already understands my wishes and it is God's "good pleasure to give" me the kingdom, as Jesus said, and then why must I ask? When I request people to pray for Carol, what do I really want them to do? I want them to hold her in their consciousness and see her healed when they connect with their Divine. But how they can do that or how I can do that, I don't know! I am certain of one thing: the prayer I grew up with is not my answer.

Attending a Baptist Church in Southeastern Kentucky, I was that "little boy" Carol Ruth spoke of. Church on Sunday morning, stretching into the afternoon, and another service that evening, lasting into the night, featured long, long prayers that rivaled the hell-fire and brimstone jeremiads of the great Puritan ministers centuries ago. On Wednesday nights, the church devoted the entire evening to "prayer meeting," where everyone, including me, stood and acknowledged our sins and shortcomings and pleaded with God, somewhere up in the sky, to take pity and forgive us so that we could go to Heaven where we would walk the streets of gold with Him forever (after we died, of course, which we hoped wouldn't happen soon). If I was eloquent enough, or loud enough, or pitiful enough, maybe God would hear me and answer my plea.

Sometimes I hit the right note or, perhaps, I caught God in a good mood and my requests would be granted. Many times, however, God did not accede to my pleas, so I must have prayed incorrectly or have sinned and fallen out of God's favor. As a teenage boy, I often felt that I had done something wrong, maybe it wasn't an evil deed, just a bad thought, usually about girls (lustful thoughts were the same as sinful acts). Instead of easing my pain, my prayers either increased my sense of guilt or made me aware of some new transgression to worry about. I kept trying to learn how to "pray right" and "live right," but the church elders I consulted never really explained to me how I could do that. My feelings of guilt reached the absurd when I took my girlfriend to see Walt Disney's "Lady and the Tramp" at the local theater. I didn't enjoy the movie because I could not quiet my internal voice which was shouting, "Shame! Shame! You have given in to worldly pleasures." The elders apparently knew what "worldly pleasures" were, but they couldn't or wouldn't explain them to me so I could avoid them and be "good." A short time later I accepted that I could never achieve the impossible standard the church expected of me and I demanded of myself. For the next twenty years I considered myself an agnostic. Oh, yes, I remember the pleading, begging, guilt-inducing prayer, but I can't believe this was what

Carol Ruth intended.

Not finding comfort in the prayer I grew up with, my thoughts shift to Carol Martha and our time in Illinois. The climatic and cultural change from California's mild weather and tolerant attitudes to southern Illinois' harsh weather and often blatant homophobia and racism were shocking to us. Six weeks after our arrival a tornado warning sent us to the basement with my visiting mother, who was recovering from surgery. The tornado cleanly removed the second story from a brick home less than two miles away. Our second winter there, temperatures dropped to twenty-five degrees below zero with a wind chill factor of fifty below. I told Carol I never again wanted to live where weather reports included "wind chill factor" or "heat index."

After about three months, Carol found a job at a counseling center in a neighboring town. Since she came from California, the agency assumed she could deal with "them" and assigned her the African-American or gay and lesbian clients who came in seeking therapy. She gladly accepted her new clients as people fully equal in

God's eyes. I'm sure these people benefited more from working with this loving rookie counselor than they would have with the experienced, prejudiced therapists.

We spent our first anniversary in a bed-and-breakfast inn in Elsah, a small town on the Mississippi River. Unlike the previous Valentine's Day on the beach in seventy degree weather, Elsah had snow. We had a wonderful weekend, which included our first view of bald eagles in the wild. The Mississippi River had frozen over as far south as Elsah and the eagles came to the edge of the frozen river to feed. Hundreds gathered in trees along the river and periodically swooped down to grab an unwary fish. We were both thrilled.

Our time in Illinois brought us even closer together. We especially enjoyed being near Saint Louis, with its concerts, shows, excellent restaurants and Cardinal baseball. I also discovered I liked researching and writing history better than teaching it. But we both were eager to return to California to be near our family and where Carol could complete her licensing requirements. My memories of Illinois make me smile, but the smile fades as I return to the present and think about Tuesday.

When Carol Ruth suggested prayer, maybe she meant the prayer that Jesus taught. As a young teenager, the last thing I did at night was repeat "The Lord's Prayer,"[7] including the words: "deliver us from evil" and "lead us not into temptation." Often I fell asleep before I finished. When I awoke and realized I had fallen asleep in the middle of the prayer, I felt guilty. I judged harshly the disciples who slept after Jesus asked them to stay awake with him in the Garden of Gethsemane, but I, too, fell asleep before I even finished this short prayer. Like the disciples, I had let Jesus down. Even after all these years, the "Lord's Prayer" still produces a twinge of guilt.

Perhaps Carol Ruth's Sunday lessons in January 1978 devoted to "The Lord's Prayer" will give me a

---

[7] Our Father, which art in Heaven, hallowed by Thy name. Thy kingdom come. Thy will be done in earth as it is in heaven. Give us this day our daily bread. And forgive us our debts, as we forgive our debtors. And lead us not into temptation, but deliver us from evil: For thine is the kingdom, and the power, and the glory, for ever. Amen. Holy Bible, King James Version, Matthew 6:9-13.

better understanding. For her, "Our Father, Who art in Heaven" is "the Essence of life" within each of us, not a white-bearded, old man, in flowing white robes, far off in some mysterious location in the sky as I had been taught. "Thy will be done," she explains, merely means letting go of my need to control. "Give us this Day our Daily Bread" is an invitation to realize that everything I need already exists within me. She urges me to increase my capacity to see deep inside, "behind the mind, behind the eyes," and to realize I often limit my "daily bread" with a tendency to specify the outcome or healing I desire. If I understand this correctly, then I should not be praying for Carol's healing, but give up my "answer" and simply watch Spirit moving through me. (*But I have not grown to that place, yet.*) "Forgive us our debts" is Jesus' message to love all of me, even my falling asleep before I finished the prayer. We all tend to love those parts of ourselves that we deem lovable and dislike or hate our perceived limitations, faults and shortcomings. By focusing on and strengthening my connection to God, I can forgive myself and learn to love all that I am. "Forgiving our debtors" is easy when I recognize that God is present in every person and every situation in my life. I know we are all one with God and there is no separate "debtor" to be forgiven. (*God is in this, too*). In discussing "lead[8] us not into temptation," Carol Ruth defines "temptation" as the "belief in evil, which means the belief in duality." (*She often refers to "duality" and "non-duality," these are concepts that I need to explore in depth.*) Many of us view life as entirely separate from ourselves and we focus our attention on an external "reality out there." I am "in temptation" when I believe what is happening to me is anything other than God unfolding in my life. To overcome a "belief in evil," Carol Ruth suggests living in the "NOW." No matter what happens, I must realize that I am "in the midst of Eternity—there is no beginning and no end—there is an infinity around [me], beyond [me], behind [me]." Life happens and I participate NOW. To do this, I must let go of the past and the future and stop reflecting, analyzing, comparing and judging myself and others. I

---

[8] Carol Ruth and Unity later changed the prayer from "*lead us not*" to "*leave us not in temptation*" reasoning God would not "lead" us into temptation.

can do this by being constantly aware of God's omnipresence and practice staying in the now. (*I am having a hard time not focusing on Carol's upcoming surgery and the "what-ifs" of the unknowns surrounding her condition.*) "For Thine is the Kingdom" means God's kingdom is mine, within me. As I explore my inner kingdom, I can discover "the Power," my source of strength, "And the glory," a sense of deep inner peace. "Forever" says without beginning or ending. Carol Ruth concludes, "The Lord's Prayer is an echo—it never ends. You are an echo—you never began; you are a sound—you will never end."[xxii]

One of the last things Carol Ruth wrote was a paraphrase of the prayer, published in Walnut Creek Unity's monthly bulletin "Center-point," in March 1987, the month after her death:

The Lord's Prayer

Our Father-Mother God
Who art in heaven as well as in earth
Hallowed be the sound of thy Presence
reverberating everywhere
Thy kingdom is now here come

Thy will is always being done
Not only in earth and all its activities
but also in the heaven of our aspiration
Thou art always giving us this day
our daily bread through all its
events and happenings whether
we can see through the eyes
of our will or not
And through your all consuming love
we know there is no sin
to be forgiven
thus strengthening us
to forgive those
who cannot harm us anyway
And any temptation we might stand in
is only the insecurity
of the unknown
As we wait in awe
before thy Kingdom
thy Power and
thy Glory
echoing into eternity
And infinity . . .

I can feel a new lightness even when I pray the original version, but especially when reciting Carol Ruth's "paraphrase." Experiencing "The Lord's Prayer" from both these perspectives allows me to say it without the sense of guilt. As I reflect on this prayer, I feel the sense of deep inner peace. As I repeat the prayer, however, I notice it begins to lose power for me. Followers of other religious traditions seem to find great comfort in numerous repetitions of simple prayers. Although there is Truth in this prayer, it is not my truth. I will keep searching.

My thoughts again shift to my years with Carol Martha. After two years in Illinois, I accepted a position as a historian at Vandenberg Air Force Base on the California coast, just north of Santa Barbara. We were thrilled. The Central Coast is beautiful and we would be about a four-hour drive from our children. Carol quickly found a paid internship with a local psychotherapist and volunteered at a residence for mental health clients to complete the 3,000 hours of supervised counseling needed for licensing. A few months later, she passed the difficult written and the even more rigorous oral examinations. She had achieved a goal set nearly ten years earlier: she was a licensed marriage and family therapist with a budding practice.

Although we loved Santa Maria, I hated my job. As a budget-saving measure, the Air Force had eliminated my original position while I was en route from Illinois. I moved temporarily to another history office to work for a person whom I immediately disliked and the feeling was mutual. Not wanting to test Carol's "whither thou goest" promise before she received her license, I resolved to do my best in what seemed to be an intolerable situation. Long walks together on Pismo Beach and her loving support made the situation bearable, at least temporarily. My choice soon became either move or leave history to work in Public Affairs writing short articles for the base newspaper, which I had neither the training nor the inclination to do.

Fortunately for me, a new organization at Beale Air Force Base, north of Sacramento, needed an historian. I submitted my application and was hired. Again I asked Carol to abandon the practice she had begun in Santa Maria and move to a place where she knew no one. She readily agreed.

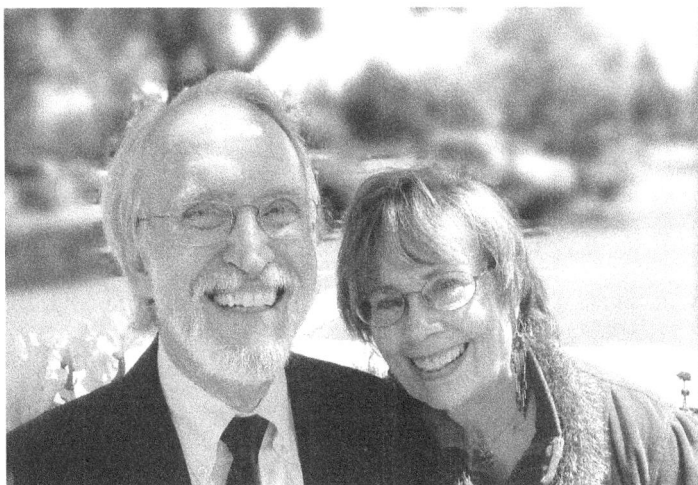

"And [Carol] said . . . whither thou goest, I will go; and where thou lodgest, I will lodge . . . "

This time I promised, "I will not ask you to move again. We will stay here and you can build a therapy practice." We quickly adapted to our new home. I loved writing history at Beale and after several months of hard work, Carol was helping people change their lives for the better. For the past seventeen years, she has been fulfilling her commitment to her "life's purpose" and doing "God's work".

My loving memories quickly give way to the thought that keeps plaguing me, "If she was doing God's work, then why would that work be interrupted or, worse yet, stopped altogether?" I don't understand. I quickly recognize this line of thinking is a waste of time. I need to find a prayer practice I can use to support her. I will study Carol Ruth's views of prayer for an answer that resonates inside me. As I do, I acknowledge that I am still seeking with my intellect, but hopefully the search will reveal a path to my heart, my intuition. As I agonize for answers, I revert to what I know best, even though some part of me knows insight will not come from my head. At least this will let me focus on something other than "What will the surgeons find when they operate on Carol? Will it be worse than what we have been told? What if they say she is beyond hope?" Seeking solutions outside myself will at least keep my mind busy.

As a young minister, Carol Ruth's beliefs were close to Charles Fillmore's. When she began her ministry in 1970, she taught prayer and meditation as a means for bringing the "unmanifested" into your life. As she grew in her ministry, her concept of prayer evolved. While continuing to teach that prayer could produce miracles "(which is no miracle but rather rightness manifested in our personal physical, emotional, mental, interpersonal lives)," she acknowledges that all conditions must be in harmony for immediate results. When God doesn't provide the instant answer we are expecting, the situation we perceive as negative could have come to us to promote our soul's growth.

Her prayer focus gradually shifts from external results to internal or spiritual benefits. Instead of concentrating on the problem, she stresses loving God with "all your heart and with all your mind and with all your soul." She believes Jesus healed by relating to the physical environment from his spiritual nature. This spiritual nature produces results not necessarily visible in the physical world. To her, being "born again" means interpreting all life from a spiritual perspective instead of using only our logic. Carol Ruth teaches that despite outward appearances my wife Carol is already whole and perfect in the mind of God. But, Carol Ruth admits, "The more I live, the more I know that I really can't spend much time with cause or how or why or finding answers to those questions."[xxiii] Interestingly, I have found "Why?" to be my least helpful question. Asking, "Why did Carol get cancer?" has no relevant answer and keeps me stuck in a quagmire of sadness, anger and an inability to act constructively. Instead, perhaps, as Carol Ruth proposes, I need to devote myself to God and trust "things will take care of themselves".

After several years as Walnut Creek's minister, Carol Ruth's thoughts on prayer continued to develop. She notes that many of us have "outgrown" our traditional religious training and move to "positive-thinking" churches that teach if we love Jesus and pray affirmatively, we will avoid pain and live happily ever after. Positive thinking also promises if we clean up our "stinking thinking," we can attract riches, relationships and good health and repel poverty, divorce and disease. Carol Ruth equates this to God's saying, "Clean up your thinking and I'll let you have control" of your life. Although asking God for specific answers seems to work for a while, eventually all the positive thinking and affirmative prayers do not produce the desired results consistently. "Haven't you tried to 'right think' your way to God in prayer?... Haven't you tried visualization, tried to get rid of judgments, tried to forgive?"[xxiv] When I don't get the answers I am seeking, my first response often is to feel guilty, as I did as a child and believing, "I must not be worthy." This also implies that I have created or attracted all painful conditions into my life. This teaching infers that if my child is sick or I lose my job or my spouse leaves or gets cancer, it is the result of my thinking. It is my fault. I refuse to let my mind go there. If someone implies that Carol or I attracted her cancer to us, my first impulse will be to punch them in the nose and say, "You attracted that to yourself."

What Carol Ruth proposes next can be shocking to Truth students. Most of our religious teachings have us trying to "figure God out" to gain control of our lives, "when the truth is *there is no control*, you are *not* in charge, there is *nothing* to understand because you don't have it within you to understand…God and God's process is larger than this, vaster, beyond the mind and its workings." She even questions Charles Fillmore's tenet that "our mind works as God's mind works," and says instead, "the real dignity, the real adulthood, the real maturity spiritually is to recognize 'I do not know—I cannot figure it out—I am not in charge—I am not in control—*God is the one responsible and I seek a way to give myself over to that Spiritual Life Force.*'" [xxv] Carol Ruth quotes Plotinus to explain how this can be done, "Let us know God Himself…by elevating our souls to Him in prayer. And the only way, truly to pray is to approach alone the one who is alone. To contemplate that one, we must withdraw into the inner soul as into a temple and there be still."[xxvi]

She also suggests that I observe the world around me. The intricacies of a flower reveal God's process and are beyond understanding. Beautiful music creates a "rush" and a "knowing" that something far greater than I is at work in the Universe. For her, stepping into that moment and merging into life relieves any sense of unfairness in our lives. She offers two steps for reaching this special moment. First, I must become as a little child, which means stop depending on my intellect to figure out the solution. Behind my mind is "a looseness that is willing to stand in awe." (*Giving up reliance on my intellect is my big challenge!*) The next step, seek God in prayer. She directs me to go within and humbly get down on my knees, either externally or internally. "That is humility. . . . That is how Abraham did it, Joseph did it, Moses did it." [xxvii]

Prayer later became the object of intense study for Carol Ruth. This convinced her to move "away from the external world's expectations to learning how to relate to my soul at an internal level." She discovered prayer has four stages. The first, "affirmation," sows a new thought in the mind. As I repeat the new thought, it will gradually move from my head into my heart. Once the message is coming from my heart, it becomes an automatic part of me. Carol Ruth describes the process as "deprogramming" myself from the "information of the world" and understanding that "all life is a matter of Spirit." Affirmations start the long process where "the message of Spirit, its concepts and values, have a chance to come from" my internal space.[xxviii]

"Denial," the second type of prayer, does not mean that what is happening to me does not exist, although some Unity ministers interpret "denial" this way. She emphasizes that by using denials I can take my "life energy" away from what I know pulls me "off center, away from Christ clarity…and allow that life energy to go in another direction." This can help remove fear and lead to the realization that nothing can hurt me.[xxix]

Next is "Prayer of the Heart," an ancient practice to move beyond my mind. By consciously bringing my attention into my heart space and repeating a prayer as simple as "I AM," I can feel a different energy. "This activity, the prayer of the heart, not only elevates consciousness and calms one's being, it is also a grounding device." If I can stay focused in the heart space and not allow my mind or emotions to "run away" with me, Carol Ruth promises "something wonderful begins to happen."[xxx]

The prayer of the heart practice can lead to the fourth type of prayer, "grace." Growing up, I believed God granted me Divine love and protection whenever I earned it. I now know God's grace is and always has been present in my life. All I have to do is recognize that presence. Living with this knowledge of constant grace can give me a sense of existing "in a cocoon of love and protection." Fear can penetrate, if it has a lesson to teach; but, "fear of fear leaves". I will no longer need to affirm, I'll be "affirmed through". I will become aware that I am being "lived through, breathed through" and it will always be there.[xxxi] I want to practice Carol Ruth Knox's 'Prayer of the Heart', but it takes time, so I will postpone that type of prayer until after Carol's surgery.

I now see prayer differently. For me, it is not about specific words or requests or pleadings or treasure mapping or affirmations or denials. There is no anthropomorphic God out in space somewhere, God is inside me. I am one with God, so my attention is directed inward. But it isn't about changing God's mind or God's image, it is about changing me. There is an answer to any question, even before the question arises, and that answer is inside. God is omniscience, omnipotence, and omnipresence. God is all knowledge, all power, and all presence. And that God exists inside me. Prayer, for me now, is reaching that internal space where I know I am connected with God and to rest quietly in that Presence listening for the "still small voice". I am still not clear, however, how to get there. I will keep trying to reach God inside me, but right now my only prayer is a prayer of thanksgiving and gratitude: "Thank you, God, for all the joys and blessings of today."

I carry this prayer as Carol and I check in at Sutter General's front desk. I have never been inside this hospital before and have some misgivings based on my previous hospital experiences. But the staff's friendliness and professionalism quickly dispel my preconceptions. Doctor Owens' nurse has already scheduled everything and the hospital staff is expecting us. The admissions clerk calls Carol's name and we move to her desk and begin to answer the myriad of questions bureaucracy deems necessary. I soon notice, however, the woman asking the questions is not an unfeeling automaton, but a real, live, feeling human being. As with our family doctor and Doctor Owens, Carol is being treated very professionally, but with loving kindness. As we finish, Carol shares with her, "I'm telling everyone today 'all the hands that touch me are the hands of God!' and you are the first." With this, the clerk stands up, gives Carol a hug, and says, "I will pray for you."

We take the elevator to the surgical floor, where a gruff-looking nurse awaits to prepare Carol for surgery. The nurse quickly disproves my first impression. Carol tells her, "I want you to know I'm telling everyone here today, 'All the hands that touch me are the hands of God!'" And this nurse, too, treats Carol with loving kindness, wrapping her in warm blankets while taking her temperature and blood pressure. When the surgical nurse comes for Carol, the prep nurse, too, hugs Carol and says, "I'll pray for you."

"Coincidentally", the surgical nurse is an ovarian cancer survivor. I kiss Carol "goodbye for now", then hear her tell the surgical nurse, "All the hands that touch me are the hands of God."

As I join our children and Greg in the surgery waiting room, I carry the prayer, "Thank you, God, for all the joy and blessings of today." Surrounded by people I love helps me feel blessed. Beth and Mellissa ask if I would like a coffee and after I say, "Yes," they walk a dozen blocks or more to find a Peet's coffee shop. Their sweet gesture makes me smile. Still, four hours pass slowly with lots of small talk and no discussion of the subject on all our minds. Finally, Doctors Owens and Beneke appear and tell us, "We removed all the cancer large enough to be removable. It went even better than we expected." He went on to explain that eighteen weeks of chemotherapy, beginning within the next couple of weeks, should kill all the remaining microscopic "spackle" (the surgeon's "medical" term for the cancer cells too small to physically remove) and make this an ovarian cancer success story.

"Thank you, God, for all the joy and blessings of

today."

About forty-five minutes later, Melvin an intensive care unit nurse, wheels Carol from the operating room recovery area. He is hesitant to stop, but I implore him to at least let us see her and let me kiss her before he hurries on. Reluctantly he does, but "only for a minute" and I think he's looking at the second-hand on his watch to make sure we don't exceed our time limit. I've never been so happy to see her face or to kiss her as I am in this moment. Too quickly, he says, "Time's up! You can see her later in the ICU!" and whisks her away.

Greg and our son and younger daughter leave after seeing Carol. Daughter Beth and I wait to get into the ICU. Shirley arrives with "comfort food," Italian salad, minestrone and pasta. Beth and I eat while Melvin connects Carol to the numerous machines, intravenous drips, and monitors that will allow nurses to constantly observe any changes in her condition. We then spend a couple of hours with Carol, who is hardly aware that we are here. I soon realize Melvin is another angel as he tends her with such professional skill together with loving kindness. To me, he is the epitome of what every nurse should aspire to.

I find great comfort in looking at her and watching her breathe. Throughout the evening I continue to give thanks for "all the joys and blessings." I also carry two other prayers or mantras.

The first Carol shared with her psychotherapy clients when their minds began to "spin out of control" with worry about what might happen in the future: "What do you know for sure, right now?" I know she is alive, the surgery went well, and her prognosis is excellent. This keeps me focused on the NOW instead of creating unhappy scenarios of what might happen in the future.

The second comes from Adyashanti, who teaches, "Let everything be as it is!" This allows me to accept Carol's cancer and to see more clearly what I can do next, instead of dwelling on "Why is this happening to us?" or "What did we do to deserve this?" I am still sad and I still cry, but I am not stuck there. I laugh and experience joy, too. It all seems surreal. I know our lives are already changed, and in ways that I can't even imagine yet.

After arriving home late tonight I e-mail our friends and family with the good news. Adding, "We all feel blessed and believe much of the success comes from the prayers around the world. Thank you so much. Keep the prayers flowing and I will let you know when she feels well enough for visitors or phone calls...We love you all very much, and thanks again for your love and support, Coy and Carol."

Later Carol acknowledges, "I feel lifted up by the prayers around the world, even from people I don't know." An interesting thought occurs to me, I have been seeking a deeper understanding of prayer. This experience will certainly give me, if not deeper understanding, at least a greater appreciation for prayer. My mind now knows prayer isn't about persuading God to cure Carol's cancer. My purpose for praying is to feel God's presence so profoundly that I can see He/She/It is already here, even in the cancer. While I haven't been able to feel that connection yet, perhaps, meditation or "Prayer of the Heart" will help me feel God's presence in my life.

Chapter 4 - The Path of Meditation

Meditation is a summoning up within oneself of a state of being that is not something to be created, but our deepest reality. You see, we don't make it up, it is in us, and we open a pathway for it to be revealed. [xxxii]

- Carol Ruth Knox

I asked for peace for myself, my family, our country and our world. The answer came: "If you will have peace, love!"

I asked for the sadness to be removed from me, my family, our country and our world. The answer came: "If you will have joy, serve!"

- Coy Cross, The Author

It's the day after surgery and I awaken early and call the intensive care unit to check on Carol. The nurse surprises me by putting Carol on the phone. Hearing her voice, I feel tears of joy and gratitude arising. She sounds wonderful, but very tired. I don't want to overtax her, so I tell her how happy I am, how much I love her, I will see her shortly, and then say "goodbye."

I remember my commitment and begin considering meditation as a conscious way to realize God. I first heard the term "meditation" in the 1960s when the

Beatles studied Transcendental Meditation (TM) with the Indian guru Maharishi Mahesh Yogi. By the mid-1970s, I knew several people who described extraordinary spiritual and psychic experiences while practicing TM. TM was "cool" and I wanted to participate, but I lived in a small town and TM centers were a city phenomenon. I took a few classes and read a few books, but, like prayer, I couldn't do it "right." When I found Unity I discovered Charles Fillmore taught meditation nearly one hundred years earlier. I continued to dabble with meditation, but never disciplined myself enough to practice regularly. Now, I have a much deeper purpose for learning to meditate. I am not trying to be "cool"; I am not looking for psychic powers; I want to know God. I will take another look at Fillmore and Unity's teachings on the subject. But that will have to wait until later today.

After breakfast, Beth and I head for the hospital. Carol is tired and sore. Melvin is back for another 12-hour shift and is carefully tending Carol and monitoring her progress. She is doing well, except when she tries to sit up her blood pressure drops dramatically to about 60/40 (normal is considered 120/80). On Doctor

Beneke's orders she will stay in the ICU at least one more day. Unlike my previous experience with ICUs, my visiting time is not limited. Beth's visit is short, she has a two-and-a-half hour drive home and she must work tomorrow. I spend the day talking with Carol when she's awake and being with her while she sleeps, leaving only to eat or use the bathroom.

While she is sleeping, I read Charles Fillmore's writings on meditation, which he defines as "continuous and contemplative thought…a steady effort of the mind to know God" with the purpose of expanding the consciousness and realizing "divine Truth". If God and man exist as spirit, Fillmore believed communication between the two must be possible or "the whole thing is a fraud". Seeking that connection, Fillmore sat in silence every night trying to "get in touch with God". Approaching this daily endeavor as a "cold, calculating business method" without enthusiasm, he continued month after month without conscious results. As the habit developed, he began to enjoy it. Eventually, he became aware of having "exceedingly realistic dreams," which he ignored at first as he continued buying and selling real estate. One day, while closing a deal on a piece of property, he remembered dreaming of this exact transaction several months before. As he paid closer attention to his dreams, he recognized them as his mode of communication from "Headquarters." He notes, "Again and again I have had mapped out the future along certain lines for months and years ahead, and the prophecies have so far never failed, although I have sometimes misinterpreted the symbols which are used."xxxiii

Fillmore believed God is Mind and our mind is our "common meeting ground." But neither "God" nor "mind" can be described, trying only limits them. "We can only say: I am mind; I know. God is Mind; He knows. Thus knowing is the language I use in my intercourse with God."xxxiv Our minds are filled with thoughts, which may be true or false. We must weigh each in "the balance of good judgment" and release all except one: "I want to know Truth, I am willing to learn. I want to express radiant health."xxxv

When Carol awakens our conversations are brief, usually limited to my telling her how beautiful she is and how happy I am her surgery went so well. Pain medications keep her responses to few words. I leave about nine p.m., promising to return early tomorrow morning, and have a late dinner at home. I spend time playing with our cat Bella, and then try meditating following Fillmore's suggestions.

But I can't get out of my head. My thoughts shift from seeking to "know the Truth" to Carol in the hospital. After a while, I give up and go to bed. Tomorrow I will see what Emilie Cady says on the subject.

Today is Thursday, two days after surgery. When I awaken, I call and talk with Carol. Her voice sounds stronger today. After breakfast and a shower, I am off to the hospital with *Lessons in Truth* in hand. Although still hurting, she is able to sit without nearly fainting. She still can't stand without her blood pressure falling well below normal. Our talks are longer as she asks if I have phoned her mom. "No, but Dave called. He is keeping Kay updated and he will be here Saturday." That brings a smile as she and Brother Dave are very close. "And, Sue is flying in today." News of her daughter's imminent arrival initiates another smile, this time even bigger.

When she sleeps, I turn to Cady. Unity gathered and published a series of Emilie Cady's talks as *Lessons in Truth* and continues to use as a basic guide to Unity principles. In the book, Cady elaborates on Fillmore's concept of "Sitting in Silence". This is not a "lazy drifting," but a "definite, waiting upon God".

If I am to sit in silence as she suggests, I withdraw bodily and mentally from the outside world after finding a time and a place where I am not likely to be disturbed. Then I take a few moments to speak directly to God - to center my mind—saying something like, "Thou abidest within me; Thou art alive there now; Thou hast all power; Thou art now the answer to all I desire." I become absolutely still, relaxing my entire body. If my mind wanders, I bring it back by saying, "It is being done; Thou art working in me; I am receiving that which I desire." Cady cautions me not to look for signs or wonders, but simply to rest in the knowledge that whatever I want is "flowing in and will come forth into manifestation either at once or a little farther on." Cady recommends closing with a prayer of thanksgiving, thanking "this innermost Presence" for hearing and answering my request.[xxxvi]

As I consider Cady's approach to meditation, Carol awakens. We talk for a bit, then it is time for her dinner. Melvin moves her to a chair and she eats several bites of Jell-O and a few more of apple sauce. She sits for nearly forty-five minutes before returning to bed. She has progressed enough to move later tonight from the ICU into a regular room. About six-thirty p.m. Sue calls, she has just landed in Sacramento and is on her way to the hospital. The news brings a large smile to Carol's face. She and Sue have a special mother-daughter bond that often allows either to know what the other is experiencing or thinking, even when they are miles apart. Sue arrives shortly and after a couple of minutes, I go to the cafeteria for coffee leaving the two of them private time together.

Later, Carol moves to a regular room near the nurses' station in the oncology surgery wing. After she is settled, I kiss her goodnight and come home. Sue opts to stay, even though it is already after eleven p.m. This represents another family-friendly change in hospital procedures; visiting hours are not limited as long as it doesn't affect the patient's recovery. This evening I try Cady's meditation suggestions, but I am not comfortable with her words. Also, her approach seems too results-oriented for me.

The days pass slowly. Carol is still sleeping a lot as she recovers. I use the time to seek a more current Unity view on meditation, so I read Eric Butterworth's ideas on the subject. He describes it as "the inward art" with an "emphasis on turning within, touching the depths of your inner self: the point where God is manifesting as you." For Butterworth, God is not someone to pray to, but a "depth of awareness and energy to pray from." Meditation provides the power that has been lacking in the concept of prayer in the many Christian churches that have dismissed meditation as a heretical practice. He suggests incorporating meditation into a "scientific prayer" by sitting quietly and relaxing; turning within and connecting with "the secret power"; then projecting this power through "an affirmation or treatment."[xxxvii]

Butterworth prefers the term "silence" over "meditation," believing this emphasizes a "state of consciousness, instead of a mental exercise." My purpose, he says, "is to recognize I am part of God. So there is no required technique. I don't need to learn a method, only to possess a desire to contact God".

Butterworth promises that God is seeking me. Within each of us at all times is a "transcendent power." By frequently quieting myself and centering on the "still point within," I become the "focus of the limitless energy of the universe… There is never a moment in your life when the guidance you desire or the creative ideas you need are not present within you, as dynamically present as the force of gravity."[xxxviii] Butterworth's thoughts resonate with me. But I have difficulty staying centered on the "still point within." After a few moments, my mind wanders; usually back to thoughts of Carol

She is making good progress, up to a point. She can sit for 30-45 minutes, but whenever she stands her blood pressure drops and she nearly faints. Today is Sunday, day five after surgery.

Dave arrived last night and Carol is really pleased to

see him. He had surgery last year. Then, while in the hospital recovering, he suffered a mild heart attack. He and Carol haven't seen each other since being together in Twin Falls for their mother's serious illness before Dave's hospitalization. Dave is still Carol's "big brother" and having him here lifts her spirits.

I talk with Maria, the "angel of mercy" who is Carol's nurse today, about her inability to stand or walk. Maria believes the pain medication could be causing the blood pressure drop. She calls Doctor Beneke and he acknowledges it's possible and orders a change to another drug. Hopefully, this will be the answer.

It's Tuesday and Dave has been with us three days now. Carol, Sue and I are all thrilled to have him here, but he must fly home this evening. We have all really enjoyed his time here. I have especially appreciated the one-on-one talks we've had. Although we have been brothers-in-law for more than twenty years, we have never before had this much time with just him and me.

Today is a good day! Doctor Beneke spent time with Carol and me this morning, checking Carol's incision, and discussing her progress. He feels she is doing extremely well. The change in medication is working. She can sit and stand without the drop in blood pressure. She will have her first solid food this evening and should be walking tomorrow. Her biggest treat, however, will be getting her hair washed later today.

But there is bad news, too. Sue and I drove Dave to the airport and stopped for coffee on the way back. We haven't had a chance to talk at length since she came home. Sue shares that Don, Carol's first husband and Sue and Michael's father, went into ICU on Tuesday the day of Carol's surgery. Sue does not know his specific diagnosis. Although Carol and Don have been divorced for more than thirty years, as parents of two children there is still a special connection between them. Sue and I decide to wait until Carol is feeling better before telling her about Don.

After we return to the hospital, I learn that angels come in different guises. When Sue and I enter Carol's room, I see immediately that she is furious. She tells us a case worker from hospital administration came into her room, awakened her, and brusquely told her she was not progressing quickly enough. Carol explained the pain medication had caused her to nearly faint each time she tried to stand, but that seems better now. The case worker responded, "Still, you are not making good progress. Perhaps we need to move you to a rehabilitation hospital." At that point, Carol was so upset she yelled at the woman to "get the #### out of my room" and then began to cry. Instead of trying to comfort or reassure her, the case worker simply left the room.

By the time Sue and I walk in Carol's tears have turned to anger. "Who does she think she is? I am making progress. Just yesterday they determined the pain medication was causing my blood pressure to drop. I am not going to a rehabilitation hospital."

I am outraged. Everyone we have dealt with in this hospital has been a living example of loving kindness and suddenly, when I am not present, a case worker acting like Nurse Ratchett (the heartless nurse in the movie *One Flew Over a Cuckoo's Nest*) appears and bullies Carol. I storm out and vent to the charge nurse, "I never want that woman in Carol's room again. More than that, I don't want anyone from administration talking to her without my being present." As I stride down the hall to "walk off my anger," I suddenly realize that woman was an angel in disguise.

Yesterday, I urged Carol to push herself harder, but she reacted, "You want me to do more than I am able. I am doing the best I can. I don't like it when you do that!" I apologized and agreed to "back off." But I was frustrated, thinking I was trying to help. "Nurse Ratchett," whatever her intent, did more to motivate Carol than I ever could. But I decide to wait a day or two before sharing my insight with Carol.

At dinner Carol eats her first solid food since surgery. We talk for a while and I leave for home. Sue stays with her mom.

At home, I consider Joel Goldsmith's "contemplative meditation" practice that promises "an experience in which we know that there is a God."[xxxix] Meditation's only purpose is to experience "God-contact or God-realization."[xl] To begin, he recommends I sit in a straight back chair, with both feet on the floor, chin in, and both hands resting in my lap. This is a natural position that can be maintained for several minutes without discomfort. Contemplative meditation includes holding a God-directed idea or question in my mind. If extraneous thoughts intrude, I'm to release them and refocus on my question. He cautions against trying to stop or blank out thinking, which is probably impossible anyway. My meditation is to be directed at the point inside where I am one with God, not towards correcting or removing any circumstance or condition.

After contemplating on an aspect or quality of God until I come to the end of my thoughts, I am then to become quiet and listen for the "still small voice." Goldsmith explains it may speak in words or an impression or a feeling or simply a deep sigh, but I will feel God's presence within me. "The moment you gain that awareness, you have made your conscious contact with God and have attained the conscious realization of your oneness with God."[xli] This practice seems easier to sustain. I can do this. I practice, but have a hard time staying focused on anything but Carol.

Today's Wednesday, the day after the "Nurse

Rachett Incident." Carol is eating solid food. Her catheter is out. The IV tube is disconnected and the needle has been removed from her arm. With aid of a walker, she walked several yards down the hallway three times and to the bathroom. She will be coming home tomorrow. Thank God for Nurse Ratchett! She helped Carol move from "Victim" to "Victor."

As I seek to develop a meditative practice that works for me, a friend suggests looking at Buddhism, since Buddhists have relied on meditation as a path to enlightenment for more than 2,500 years. Interestingly, Adyashanti, a contemporary Buddhist teacher, in his "True Meditation" or "meditative self-inquiry," advises an approach similar to Goldsmith's "contemplative meditation." Posture is not an important element for him, any comfortable position, other than lying down, is acceptable. Lying down often causes sleepiness.

I connect with the senses to anchor myself in the moment. "Through your senses, open to the whole world within and around you. This grounds you in a deeper reality than your mind." The peace and stillness I seek are already present within me. If my attention wanders, I'm to bring it back by tuning in to the senses, "what do I hear?" or "what do I feel?" Then, I allow everything to be as it is. Next, I ask a "spiritually powerful question," for example "who or what am I?" This directs my attention inward, deeper than the thinking mind, because this question cannot be answered by the intellect.

I start by eliminating what I am not. If I can observe my body, then I must be more than my body. The same is true for thoughts, beliefs, feelings and ego-personality. Following this reasoning, Adyashanta concludes "awareness" or "spirit" is my true essence: what I actually am. One gem of his teaching helps me immediately: "I let everything be as it is" becomes a powerful mantra that I have been using each time I start worrying that Carol might never fully recover or that she might die. By "letting everything be as it is" I can be consciously present in the "now" and clear on what I need to do next.

As I continue my inquiry at home this evening, I listen to tapes of my friend Carol Ruth's teachings on meditation. She believes meditation arose to satisfy an internal hunger for a deeper experience as humankind developed. "Meditation exists because human consciousness [in its earliest form] created it."[xlii] The practice can satisfy several purposes, including relaxing physically, calming an anxious mind, healing the body, experiencing other levels of consciousness, and communicating and uniting with God. She says I communicate with God though ideas, sensations, feelings, sounds, intuition and an internal "knowing." Ultimately, meditation's purpose is to "bring its fruits" back into my daily life, "I am not in this work to prepare you to become meditative so that you can disappear from the world."[xliii]

To start, Carol Ruth recommends that I be alone or in a small group, I reduce external stimuli as much as possible and assume a posture that keeps my body movements to a minimum. Then, in keeping with the ancient Buddhist practice, I am to watch my breath. Being as present with the breathing as possible, I do nothing more that notice as I breathe. My mind will undoubtedly wander. When I become aware that I am thinking of something else, I return to watching the breath. "I am not attending my breath because I think I will move closer to God that way...I am only attending my breath," she reminds me.[xliv] After becoming adept at watching the breath, I begin to relax my physical body. Starting with the soles of the feet and moving slowly from sole to arch to ankle, I'm to focus attention on each body part, in order, until I reach the top of the head, making sure I include internal organs as well as.

The breathing practice helps focus my attention and relaxation creates internal space in which to dwell. It is in the dwelling that "one has the possibility of unifying with God...of opening new, creative spaces." [xlv] She cautions that I don't go into mediation to become one with God. "We meditate as a practice and an attitude of being (versus an attitude of doing), which, at times, leads to special experiences...You use the exercises to break open new ground, but you don't know what the new ground is that you are trying to break open." [xlvi]

I now have enough information and external input to create a meditation practice that fits me based on Carol Ruth's teachings with additions from the others as well. I will develop a routine I can use when other people are in the house. I withdraw to the bedroom, where I won't be interrupted, and turn on soft music. I sit in a comfortable, straight-backed chair. My knees will no longer let me sit in a half-lotus position. I remove my shoes and let my bare feet rest on a small pillow to take the pressure off my feet and legs. I bring my attention into my body by focusing on the five senses: I ask, "What do I taste?" and then allow myself to taste deeply; "What do I smell?" and I take in even the most subtle smells, scents and aromas. I continued with hearing and seeing. The answer to "What do I feel?" takes longer, because I start with feeling my feet on the pillow and gradually move to the ankles, legs, butt, back, and then through the rest of the body. If I am anxious or my mind is especially active, I focus on each part of the entire body. Other times, when I feel centered, I start with the body and then soon move directly to the breath. As I attune to my breath, I don't try to control or change it, I simply watch it. When I feel I am totally present with my breath, then I introduce my question or thought. Right now I want to move from believing to knowing God exists and experiencing God within me. I have a "head answer," but I am seeking a "heart answer."

I sit the first thing in the morning, immediately after rising, and again just before going to bed in the evening. Sitting twice a day deepens my experience. So far, meditation has brought me greater peace and acceptance than I have known before. I have also had some profound insights that seem to come from a wisdom far greater than mine. Last night while sitting in mediation, I asked for peace for myself, my family, our country and our world. The answer came: "If you will have peace, love!" I asked for the sadness to be removed from me, my family, our country and our world. The answer came: "If you will have joy, serve!" I am still searching for "God is in this, too." Maybe the answer has already come, but so subtly that I have missed it.

Thursday, June 11, Carol is home. Step One, the surgery to remove the cancer and her initial recovery, is done. She will have three to four weeks to regain strength and then Step Two, the chemotherapy regimen, will begin.

Right now we have to establish a routine to care for her needs at home. I join the local Costco and buy a rice cooker, a George Foreman grill, a juicer, and other small appliances that will make fixing nutritious meals easier. Fortunately, I retired a couple of years ago, so I have the time to be her caregiver. I gladly accept that I will be the "chief cook and bottle-washer" for the next several months. Thanks to meditation I have the insight that helping her heal is a privilege and a gift that has been given me. I have an opportunity to demonstrate my love for her by serving.

I thank God every day for the wonderful care and the loving kindness she received from everyone at the hospital and for the love and support from our family and friends. We are truly blessed. "Thank God for all the joys and blessings of today!"

Meanwhile, I will continue my inquiry. Perhaps the key is to have spiritual practice in place before the need arises. I just had two new insights as I am developing a meditation practice: first, feeling like "I am not doing it right" is reverting back to my childhood and believing I have to be perfect, which is a reflection of an ego that thinks I can be perfect; second, any method I use to contact God is the right practice for me. An omnipresent, omniscient God will understand. In the meantime, I do feel more inner peace and more capable of being consciously present with Carol.

I am looking for something to help me immediately see "God in this, too," but there may not be a "quick fix." Carol Ruth teaches "Practicing the Presence" through the "Prayer of the Heart" is a path for transformation. After several years of practice and study she made this the subject of her doctoral dissertation. I believe this, added to my mediation and prayer practices, will help me experience God more deeply. I will study her writings and Sunday messages to see why she valued this so highly.

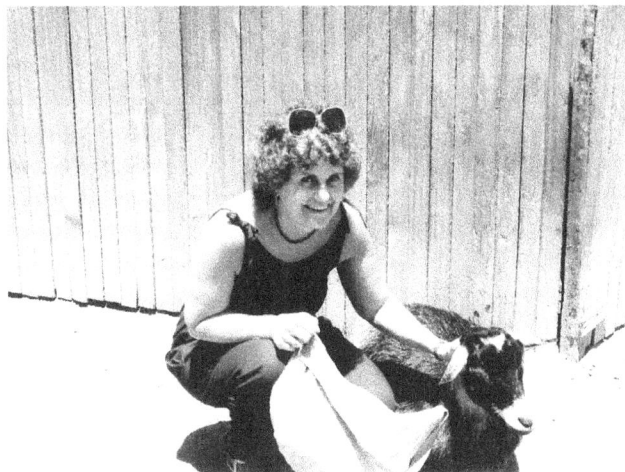

This picture was taken one of the last days Carol Ruth Knox and I spent together. We talked while enjoying the San Diego Zoo during a break from a conference in 1986. She was one of the greatest teachers I ever had. She saw God everywhere.

While at the zoo, Carol Ruth was delighted by a baby orangutan. She commented to the lady next to her, "Isn't it wonderful. These are our closest relatives."

The woman responded, "Not if you believe God, they're not." Then she stalked off.

Carol Ruth, taken aback, said to me, "She questioned my belief in God." Laughing, I responded, "That is what I find so funny." Carol Ruth, one of my greatest teachers, saw God everywhere, even in the woman, who questioned Carol Ruth's belief. We had quite a chuckle over this and it remains a great memory for me.

Chapter 5 - Practicing the Presence

Whenever a person goes through trauma or crisis, there has to be a way to put meaning into it, so that you can live with yourself for the rest of your life. xlvii

- Carol Ruth Knox

Instead of coming to save humanity from sin, Jesus [came] as a guide who opens the individual's access to spiritual understanding. Such awareness of illusion and enlightenment, and its availability to each human being, is the heart of the Prayer of the Heart. xlviii

- Carol Ruth Knox

Carol has slowly built up her stamina and strength by walking every day during the month since her surgery. Today, July 2, she has her first appointment with Doctor Stacy D'Andre, her oncologist. Stacy stopped and introduced herself before Carol left the hospital, but I have not yet met her. As we wait in the Oncology waiting area, I notice people of various ages, races, ethnicities and economic backgrounds. Cancer is an equal opportunity disease; it does not discriminate between old and young, male and female, black and white, rich or poor.

Dennis, a nurse's aide from Doctor D'Andre's office, escorts us back to a small room where he checks Carol's weight and takes her blood pressure and temperature. As Dennis finishes, Doctor D'Andre and Lisa, her nurse, come in. Stacy is young, dark-haired, pale-skinned and cute. She reminds me of Winona Ryder, although she doesn't really look like the actress. But more importantly, she is very sharp, very competent and very compassionate. For the next hour she explains Carol's chemotherapy regimen and schedule and answers our questions.

There will be six three-week cycles beginning on July 14. During Cycle I Carol will receive chemo through her IV (intravenous) port on Tuesday followed the next day by a Neulasta injection to stimulate white cell production. Each Monday the laboratory will draw blood to check her white and red cell count and other blood chemistry. Every third Monday, just prior to her appointment with Doctor D'Andre, the lab will check her CA-125 level, which reflects the ovarian cancer antigens present in her body. Beginning with Cycle II, she will undergo the IV chemo treatment on Tuesday and then check into the hospital on Wednesday for an overnight stay and two liters of chemo injected directly into her abdomen through the IP (intraperitoneal) port. Throughout the night she will be turned periodically to ensure the chemicals reach all the organs in her lower abdomen.

Stacy answers our questions directly, while reassuring us that Carol has a good chance for recovery. "Yes, the chemo is difficult, but we have learned a lot and we will give you medication to minimize the pain." "Yes, you will lose your hair, but it will grow back." "Yes, you will experience nausea, but we have medication that will keep it from becoming unbearable." "The first days after chemotherapy will be difficult, but you will gradually feel better after about a week. Our goal is for you to have more good days than bad days." As Stacy is talking, she is making notes covering the details of Carol treatment plan. Lisa is creating the extensive schedule that will govern our lives for the next several months. After Stacy has answered all our questions, she gives us her notes and Lisa hands us Carol's schedule. Stacy then hugs Carol and tells her if she has any questions or concerns to call and either she or Lisa will get back to her with an answer. We leave feeling confident that Doctor D'Andre is exactly the right person to shepherd Carol through this next phase of her recovery.

During the brief period leading up to Carol surgery and then her ten-day hospital stay, I focused on staying consciously present with her. This past month we both practiced "being in the moment." For example, "Now we are walking down to the first bench. Now we are resting and having a drink of water. Now we are walking back home." "What do we need to do right now?" We do not allow thoughts of "what if" to stay in our minds.

We create a routine, governed primarily by her medication schedule, designed to make sure she gets plenty of rest and as much exercise as she can tolerate. Each day breakfast is at eight a.m., lunch at noon, and dinner at five-thirty p.m. She has a snack with her evening meds just before bedtime. There is another snack and more meds at three-thirty to four a.m. With my limited cooking skills, I prepare nutritious food, which I supplement with take-out from our favorite restaurants: the Blue Nami and Thai Basil. Workers at both places ask about Carol each time. Again, I am aware of the loving kindness surrounding us. Soon after she came home, we began a game-a-day Cribbage tournament for "The Championship of the Whole World." We have played twenty-seven games so far.

I have also been an uncompromising gate-keeper for visitors. I only allow our family and a couple of her closest friends to see Carol and then only after grilling them about colds, flu or anything else that might hinder her progress. I have probably hurt some people's feelings, but she has to be as strong as possible to confront chemotherapy.

In the evening, while Carol is resting, I study Carol Ruth Knox's lessons on practicing the presence of God. To see God in my experience of Carol's cancer, I must reach a deeper place within myself. In 1977 Carol Ruth underwent a "very powerful spiritual experience, which had no definition, no guidelines, no maps whatsoever" and she immediately began searching for its meaning. She spent the next eight years poring through accounts by Saint Theresa of Avila, Julian of Norwich, Saint John of the Cross, the *Philokalia* and an estimated 150 other Christian and pre-Christian saints seeking answers. She concluded practicing the presence of God through constant prayer will awaken a "direct experience of God."[xlix] Joel Goldsmith agreed, "Now I saw that the principle of life, the secret of all successful living, was making God a part of my very consciousness, something which Paul describes as praying without ceasing."[1]

But how does one, or more importantly, how can I pray constantly, without ceasing? It seems that there are only a few minutes left at day's end even for study and meditation. How then can I devote all my time to prayer? Although I'm busy with household chores, doctor's appointments, laboratory appointments, cooking healthy food that Carol can eat, and a host of other things, my search for a deeper meaning for Carol's cancer is too important to overlook any possibility. I'll study Goldsmith and Carol Ruth's writings and listen to her workshop on the subject, perhaps I can find some answers.

Meanwhile, it's July 14 and Carol and I arrive at the infusion center ready for her first chemotherapy appointment. But we have a concern. Her abdomen is distended nearly as much as before her surgery. As the nurse begins the preliminary medications that will prevent the more severe reactions to the cancer drugs, Carol asks her about the distention. The nurse agrees to call Doctor D'Andre. The nurse soon returns with the news that Doctor D'Andre has ordered the chemotherapy to stop and scheduled a CT scan to check for visible signs of lingering cancer. Chemotherapy is postponed until next Tuesday.

The CT scan shows no new cancer, but a considerable buildup of fluid in Carol's abdomen. Doctor D'Andre scheduled an appointment for another doctor to drain the fluid. So we spend a couple of hours today, Friday the 17th, while a doctor drains three-and-a-half liters (nearly one gallon) of fluid from her abdomen. But we still don't know the cause. Carol and I joke that she has a new weight-loss program—she lost twelve pounds in one day.

The nurse, who attends today, says Carol reminds her of a beloved therapist the nurse had seen in Redding, California. She takes Carol's business card and promises to contact her when she resumes practicing psychotherapy. This is a huge boost for Carol's self-image. She considers all such "coincidences" as "God winks."

Doctor Beneke calls later in the afternoon and explains the fluid buildup. The extensive scraping during her surgery caused her abdominal tissues to weep fluid. This is a normal reaction to such an invasive procedure. Neither the CT scan nor the lab tests reveal anything new. There is no residual cancer.

While waiting for Cycle I, I look first at Joel Goldsmith's thoughts on practicing the presence. He cautions "no one can ever reach God with conscious thinking: God can only be reached through a receptive state of consciousness...If we live in meditation, giving sufficient periods to maintaining our contact with the Presence, ...at any moment that there is a necessity or need, God will speak to us."[li] Goldsmith reminds me that God is always present within me, so there is no need to seek God anywhere else. He promises if I persistently hold the thought "The kingdom of God is within me" several times each day, eventually "An experience takes place—it may be a feeling of warmth; it may be a feeling of release; it may be a voice in the ear;

but it is something that takes place within, and we, within ourselves, know that we have had a visitation of the Christ."[lii]

It's July 21 and the chemotherapy treatments begin today. After the drama surrounding the aborted first chemo cycle, today's actual infusion is uneventful. Last week's practice run prepared Carol for today and she feels less anxious. The loving kindness continues. She asks for and receives a bed in a private room, instead of a lounge chair in an open area. The nurse's aide, who checks her weight, blood pressure and temperature, makes her feel cared for by wrapping her in warm blankets. The nurse, who administers the cancer drugs, explains what she is doing at each step, what the drug is, what it is for, what Carol will feel, what she can expect in the next several days, and anything she should be aware of. We sit talking at times, reading a bit, simply cherishing that we are together, and being consciously present. Five hours later, we stop by Jamba Juice on our way home to celebrate a successful day.

The single Neulasta injection to stimulate white cell growth on Wednesday seems minor in comparison to yesterday's chemotherapy and the medications helped minimize the pain. Later this evening, however, the bone-deep ache from today's injection begins. For immediate impact, the Neulasta is more painful than the chemotherapy. Although the chemotherapy side-effects do not begin for about two days after her infusion, the nausea and neuropathy (tingling and pain in her fingers and toes) soon have a profound effect. A nightly foot massage provides limited relief, but she enjoys being touched.

Carol Martha quickly learns she must take the anti-nausea medication before she starts feeling nauseous. If she waits until she experiences symptoms, it is too late. She also has increased the pain medication to be able to tolerate the pain. Thank God, she is responsible for her own medication regimen and she is so considerate that she lets me get several hours of uninterrupted sleep.

With no appetite, she eats only because she needs the nourishment. The least effort requires all her energy; and, she generally feels like "I've been run over by a truck." Gradually, the nausea subsides, her appetite and energy level improve and we can walk about a quarter of a mile with frequent rest stops. We have also found added benefits from our "Championship of the Whole World" Cribbage tournament: shuffling and dealing the cards exercises her fingers and helps offset the neuropathy that comes with chemotherapy, and counting points aids in counteracting "chemo brain," our "medical term" for muddled thinking that often accompanies chemotherapy.

As she rests, I return to practicing the presence. Carol Ruth's approach differs from Goldsmith's in that she uses prayer instead of meditation to practice the presence. This is not ordinary prayer, but "The Prayer of the Heart," which became her dissertation topic. I took Carol Ruth's workshop on "Prayer of the Heart" in 1984 and I read her dissertation; however, I have long since let the details and the practice fade from memory.

This ancient practice began about one hundred years after the death of Jesus with a group of dedicated Christian men, who withdrew into the Egyptian desert seeking a direct experience of God. These "Desert Fathers" lived alone in small caves, as hermits in community with other hermits. Also called Hesychasts or "those who are in pursuit of the silence together," they often spent years without speaking to another person, even fellow community members. Carol Ruth describes this as a "living silence" in which the Desert Fathers carried this prayer ongoing, in their hearts, with full devotion, while watching the prayer's work within. They literally prayed without ceasing.

I have often thought it would be easier to lead a spiritual life if I could withdraw into an ashram or live in a retreat center or even a small cabin in the mountains or by the sea. But I have a family and responsibilities and one can only "retreat" for so long, then "the world" pulls me back in. No, I must find a practice that includes being with Carol and living my life. I do trust Carol Ruth. So with her promise that the "Prayer is a vehicle for transformation" and that "the dark night be worn, the weaknesses addressed, the sins used for learning and steps toward love, and the pain realized as a purging fire of renewal," I reintroduce myself to the Prayer of the Heart.

We are ready for Cycle II. At yesterday's appointment with Doctor D'Andre, Stacy decided to change chemo drugs to reduce the neuropathy. If allowed to continue, the condition could become permanent. She also explained that Carol's lab results showed a CA-125 level of 72, reflecting the continued presence of ovarian cancer antigens in the blood. Normal is below 35, prior to surgery Carol's was over 1,000 and before her first chemo cycle it was over 80. So the chemo is working. Another piece of good news, this cycle will not include the harsher intraperitoneal infusion (IP treatment) directly into the abdomen, which requires an overnight stay in the hospital. And, her white cell count is high enough that she won't need the Neulasta shot.

Each week we receive copies of all the lab reports and are becoming amateur experts on blood chemistry. We pore over each report looking at red cell count, white cell count, CA-125, and even trace minerals such as magnesium, comparing this week's results with last week's. Any change we don't understand or that causes concern prompts a call to Doctor D'Andre. Either she or Lisa or Laura, D'Andre's physician's assistant, always phone back with explanations and reassuring answers.

Cycle II is similar to Cycle I. Again, Carol is in the private room, wrapped in warm blankets. The nurse and nurse's aide are personable, asking questions about our family and answering our inquiries about their families, but always with a professional air. There is casual chatter, but never a sense of casual care. Every person we encounter is working here because they want to, because they have asked to and most have many years experience. This is very reassuring to both Carol and me. We talk about our children and her mother and what we will have for dinner tonight. We don't talk about what the future might hold. In fact, we don't even consider what we'll have for dinner tomorrow night. We are present to today. The new drug takes less time to administer, so we are soon enjoying our Jamba Juice on our way home.

I have regularly called or e-mailed family and friends of Carol's progress, but today, two weeks after her second chemotherapy treatment, she feels well enough to update everyone herself. Her message both touches me deeply and makes me smile. She writes, "I am flooded with your words, love, caring and encouragement. Please know that they help carry me through the hardest days. Thank you for them and your ongoing wishes and prayers." Reading this causes tears to flow. Then I smile as I continue reading, "The luxurious locks (I never really had) are about gone now, along with extra pounds, so I'm a slimmer, less hairy, version of myself. I'm wishing for thick, curly, auburn locks by Christmas. Meanwhile, wigs are not my thing. Rather, I'm choosing colorful babushkas (scarves)—with earrings, of course!" Her concluding sentences reaffirm the wisdom and beauty of this woman I married, "I want you to know I'm practicing 'Being in the Now' each day and it carries me through what that day presents. Being in the moment, something I have counseled for years, has become my life." And with that my tears began again.

I return to Carol Ruth's messages. Today, I learn my desire to see God in Carol's cancer "comes from God." So I will have divine assistance in my search. My first step in practicing the presence is to focus my entire attention in my heart. This "heart" is not my internal organ, but my spiritual heart at the center of my being, "penetrating through the body and emanating from it."[liii]

To do this, I envision moving my attention from behind my eyes, down through the back of my throat, to a point beneath my sternum about two inches above the bottom of my ribcage. Carol Ruth acknowledges that the mind "accustomed...to external entertainment and chatter" will become "bored unless given something to do." To overcome the boredom, she suggests I repeat the Jesus Prayer, "Lord Jesus Christ, Son of God, have mercy upon me," while maintaining my attention in my heart. The Desert Fathers prayed this prayer nearly two thousand years ago and it has been in constant use ever since. The recitation is easy. The challenge is to repeat the prayer constantly with the attention in the heart, as the Desert Fathers did, but while living "in the world."[liv] Carol Ruth assuages my concern about praying constantly, "The truth is that you will only do it as much as you can and that will be your constant."[lv]

Like many "New Thought" adherents, I react to what sounds like the pleading prayers I said as a child. But for Carol Ruth these words signify something different. "Lord Jesus Christ" refers not to Jesus the man, but to universal Christ principle within each of us. "Son of God" applies not only to Jesus, but to everyone, including me. The statement "have mercy on me!" is not asking a judgmental God to think kindly of me; instead I am saying, "I stand in awe before this amazing adventure."[lvi]

Carol Ruth cautions the purpose of practicing the presence and The Prayer of the Heart is not to make my life easier or "better," but to experience God directly. "Along the way, one must face totally the inner darkness within himself; and, wonderfully and mysteriously, not only let go of self, but also see himself interconnected with all people as if of one body." [lvii]

The practice, although simple, is intense and not easy. First, I consciously bring my attention into my spiritual heart at the center of my being and keep my focus there no matter what else I may be doing. Then I constantly repeat "Lord Jesus Christ, Son of God, have mercy on me!" Whether I am cooking dinner, cleaning the bathroom, talking with Carol or being with her during chemotherapy, my focus is in my heart and my internal dialogue is the Jesus Prayer. Carol Ruth promises this practice will teach me "things which in no other way will [I] ever learn." [lviii]

Summer is ending, meanwhile, and Cycle III ushers in September. Preparation for this cycle included another CT scan last week, which came back clear. Doctor D'Andre had great news at Carol's appointment yesterday. First, she will not be undergoing the harsh IP treatments. Stacy explained these would cause the neuropathy to be "ten times worse" and could cause permanent damage. But, and more importantly, Carol doesn't need them. The two IV cycles have worked so well her CA-125 is now within the normal range at 19 (anything below 35 is normal). Doctor D'Andre also informed us that such immediate and positive response to chemotherapy bodes well for Carol's remaining cancer-free. Carol and I both cried joyous tears and hugged Stacy. I find myself crying much more easily lately and many are tears of joy.

Cycle III and Carol again gets the private room. The aide wraps her in warm blankets and takes her vital signs. The nurse explains what the chemicals are, the order they will be administered and what Carol can expect. Although a different nurse has administered the chemotherapy each time, they are all caring professionals. As the nurse prepares Carol, I have a hard time watching, so I go for coffee. When I return, the needle is inserted in the port and the first of the fluid is flowing. Our conversation today is upbeat and we are almost giddy over the good news from yesterday.

But we both know there are still hard days ahead. We have come to expect Carol will feel good the rest of today. By tomorrow evening, the neuropathy will be very painful and she will need pain meds to cope. After her first cycle, she suffered severe nausea. Now she prevents that by taking anti-nausea medication before she gets sick. The first week following chemotherapy is the worst. Week two gradually gets better. By week three, her energy and appetite improves. We have also noticed that each cycle is a little harder and the overall effect of the chemo is cumulative. But, with Cycle III, she is half-way through.

Staying "in the moment" allows us to appreciate the so-called "little" things that are the most important gifts of all. We have just had such a gift. I have always loved Carol's hair, whether she wore it long, short, up, down, curly or straight. It is a beautiful soft brown, with very little gray even though she is 68 years old. We have known from the beginning that chemotherapy would cause her to lose her hair. But even when it began falling out, she was reluctant to have it cut. Tonight a long hair lodged in her eye and we had a very difficult time removing it. She decided it was time and she wanted no one but me to cut what was left of her hair. I used my small electric beard-trimming clippers that she gave me to remove the last traces of her beautiful hair. We were both surprised to discover this was one of the most intimate moments either of us has ever experienced and one we will cherish forever.

Carol's appointment with Doctor D'Andre, prior to Cycle IV, includes more good news. Her CA-125 continues to drop and is now 9. When Carol asked if this meant she was cured, Stacy responded, "It is too soon to talk about cure. We can use the term 'remission' at this point." The actual infusion experience is again filled with warm blankets and loving kindness. But there is a reality check. A student nurse accompanies Susan the attending RN. With Carol's permission, Susan explains the infusion procedure to the student, including the need for protective gloves, gown and face-shield, "the chemicals we are injecting are extremely poisonous and you don't want to risk getting it in your eyes or on your skin." That is sobering to hear, although we are already aware of the hazards. The infusion is soon over and we're off to Jamba Juice.

The steadily improving CA-125 numbers and Stacy's statement of "remission" proves to be a two-edged sword. Although we are ecstatic that the chemo is working, Carol is finding the increasing pain and fatigue more difficult to endure. "If I am in remission and the CA-125 readings are normal, why do I have to continue this ordeal? I don't think I can do two more rounds."

Although my inner voice is saying, "You can't do that. We have gone through too much for you to quit now. You have to finish," I know it is not up to me. I am committed to honoring her right to make her own decisions. I love her, but it is her life and she must be in charge. I respond, "Sweetheart, it is always your decision. Let's get through this time and then talk with Doctor D'Andre at your next appointment. I will support you in whatever you decide."

During my quiet moments early in the morning and

late at night, I continue meditating twice each day. This brings me peace and renewed inner strength. Throughout the day, as often as I can remember, I repeat the Jesus Prayer. The main effect I feel is that it keeps me focused on something other than Carol's cancer.

As we approach her next oncology appointment, these last three weeks have been extremely difficult. Objectively, all signs indicate the chemotherapy is killing the cancer cells and Carol is in remission. Subjectively, she feels like "crap": the pain and tingling in her fingers and toes is hard to bear and affects her dexterity; her white blood count is near zero and she contracted a painful urinary tract infection; her red blood count is low so she has no energy. Although I encourage her to keep in mind how well she is doing and talk of the love and prayers of people around the world and discuss how we will have so much to celebrate this Thanksgiving, it has little effect. Her endurance and resolve are nearly exhausted. I don't tell her, but I am bone-tired, too.

Thank God for Stacy D'Andre! At Carol's preinfusion appointment, she shares with Stacy the extent of her side-effects and her reluctance to endure two more cycles of chemotherapy. Stacy proposes changing to Gemzar, a drug with reduced side-effects, and dividing the infusions into two parts spaced a week apart. More than ever, Carol so wants to live, not only for herself, but for me, our children, her mother and brother, and all the family and friends who have supported us. Adding to her determination, we have learned Don, her children's father, is terminally ill with brain and lung cancer. This news inspired a renewed determination that Mike and Sue would not lose both parents at the same time. She agrees to the new regimen and to finishing the last two cycles. I feel like we have crossed a huge hurdle. This was a life-or-death moment and she has chosen to live. Thank God for Doctor D'Andre! With the new routine, Cycle V goes smoothly.

I continue practicing the presence, but without dramatic results. I remember Carol Ruth saying, "Do ongoing prayer in the heart to assist in your evolutionary expansion. The only thing I really have to say is 'do the work! Make a commitment to do the work.'"[lix] Okay,

okay, I will "do the work" knowing full well this is a lifetime commitment. As with meditation and prayer, I expect any changes to be internal and a gradual process. This is not about instant enlightenment. It is about realizing God's presence in all things, including Carol's cancer.

Today is November 11, Armistice Day, a day to commemorate the end of World War I, "The War to End All Wars" and a fitting day for Carol to finish her chemotherapy. She just had her "last blast of the nasty Neulasta" and that concludes the chemo regimen. We are both exhausted. But, now the healing can truly begin. There is joy in River City tonight; Mighty Carol has stuck it out!

Interestingly, yesterday's final round of chemo had its own drama. As the nurse prepared her for the infusion, he nonchalantly added, "And we will be giving you two units of blood today." Both Carol and I did a double-take and told him, "No one mentioned her receiving blood." Within ten minutes, Laura, Doctor D'Andre's nurse practitioner, arrived from her office two blocks away. She explained Doctor D'Andre had ordered the transfusion because Carol's red blood count was very low. Laura also assured us the blood supply was safe and that she would not hesitate accepting blood herself, if needed. Feeling more at ease, Carol agreed to take the blood. Since each unit requires about two hours to infuse, Carol could receive the blood today with her Neulasta shot.

When I went to schedule the transfusion, however, there was no time in today's schedule. The nurse suggested coming back tomorrow or Friday. I was so tired and stressed at that point I felt like sitting down on the floor and crying, but I didn't. I asked if there was not some alternative. She thought for a moment and replied the blood was already cross-matched, so they could give it immediately after the chemotherapy, if Carol could tolerate the added time. I talked with Carol and she, too, wanted to get it over with and agreed to have the transfusion after her chemo.

Nine-and-one-half hours later, we headed for home, too exhausted to stop at Jamba Juice. On the way home, Carol said, "I so appreciate Cork (our son Coy III) and the other selfless people who donate blood. They made it possible for me to receive the blood I need to continue my healing."

Now, with the cancer in remission, she can start recovering from the chemotherapy's effects. We are eagerly anticipating Thanksgiving, my favorite holiday, and Christmas with our family. The "Championship of the World" score is 59 for Carol and 70 for me. I must confess to shamelessly taking advantage of her "chemo-brain" to build-up a lead. But joy and pain are both present—Don died last Wednesday.

I realize Carol Ruth's Prayer of the Heart will not produce the immediate insight I'm seeking. It is a life-long practice. Perhaps her thoughts on non-duality will provide some help I can use now.

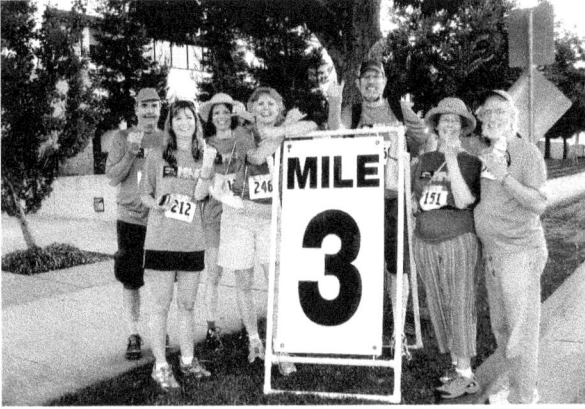

Team Carol at the Ovarian Cancer Walk in 2010 after finishing her chemo therapy.

Her strength had returned enough for her to complete the 5K walk, even though the temperature was well over a hundred degrees. People along the route turned on sprinklers and Carol did not hesitate to run through them. This is so typically Carol, making us all laugh. She moves through life with background music. During chemo, the music went away, but on this day, the music was back.

When someone close to you has a serious illness, the patterns of support become obvious. Again we are grateful for the support of family, friends and our greater community.

Chapter 6 - Non-Duality

I have only one message to offer and that is Non-duality. . . . But I don't know how to share that. I must find a way to help them take that on and challenge themselves to become single-eyed and non-dualistic.[lx]

- Carol Ruth Knox

The interesting paradox is that out of the chaos of cancer comes order and yet out of the order of recovery comes the chaos of redoing life. And, the thread of non-duality exists in both.

- Carol Martha Cross

Non-duality, Carol Ruth Knox's "one message," is the belief that there is no right or wrong, good or bad, light or dark. We are all one with everything and everything is the unfoldment of God. It just "is." Non-duality did not originate with Carol Ruth; it has been a basis for Eastern religions for centuries. She, however, introduced it to me.

My limited spiritual background includes definite thoughts on right and wrong, good and bad. I remember being awestruck when I first heard Carol Ruth explain if God is omniscience, omnipotence, and omnipresence, then obviously everything must be God's unfoldment. I have wrestled with this thought ever since, "How can I live non-dualistically in a dualistic world?"

Today, for example, Carol said she could not endure the two and a half hour drive to our daughter Elizabeth's for Thanksgiving. Is this God unfolding? This is my favorite holiday and I have been anticipating it for the last five months. All the children and grandchildren are going to be there and I haven't seen some of them since Carol's surgery. I am so disappointed, I want to argue, bargain, encourage, and cajole to make her change her mind. But I don't. She knows how much Thanksgiving with the family means to me and I know the courage it takes for her to say she can't go. She encourages me to go, but I won't leave her. I have to accept "this is what is."

Carol Ruth reminds me that living in a dualistic world is difficult and leads to the perspective of good guys in white hats battling desperadoes in black ones, of The Force against Darth Vader, who invites me, along with his son Luke, to "come over to the dark side." "Consequently, we are forever living out the battle of polarities, continually jumping from one opposite to the other,"[lxi] trying to ensure we have only Godly thoughts, anything less is evil. This returns me instantly to boyhood and my internal struggle to always be good and have thoughts worthy of Jesus. Carol Ruth seemingly speaks directly to me saying, "The process forces us to act out an exorcism. . . . It becomes intensely painful because we feel compelled to get rid of the [wrong] for the [right] to survive."[lxii] I know this struggle well.

Dualistically, I immediately want to label Thanksgiving with the family as "good" and not attending as "bad." By Thanksgiving Day I have shifted and accept "what is": Carol is not strong enough to travel to San Jose. Sue joins us at home and we start a new tradition: tacos instead of turkey. We have a wonderful day and I am truly thankful. Carol is here with me and a few months ago I wasn't sure she would be. I also tell myself "Christmas is in five weeks. The family will gather at Mellissa's and she lives only one and a half hours away. Surely Carol will be well enough to travel by then."

But first she has to be "de-ported," which in this case means Doctor Beneke taking out the chemotherapy ports that he installed during her initial surgery. He completes the simple procedure during Carol's follow-up appointment four days before Christmas. Her recovery is going well. An appointment with Doctor D'Andre confirms Carol's CA-125 is 6.2 and all her other counts are within the normal range. Carol's hair is starting to grow back, her appetite is improving and she is walking farther and at a faster pace than just a couple of weeks ago. Stacy tells us to expect recovery from chemotherapy to take about as long as the therapy itself. So we are expecting Carol to take about six months to return to "normal"; although, I am starting to realize it will be a "new normal."

Christmas does not go as I had hoped either. Not wanting to expose Carol to colds, flu, or other maladies schoolchildren often carry, we have not seen the grandchildren in several months. But Carol still does not feel well enough to make the trip to Mellissa's. My longing for a "grandchildren fix" is so strong I attend the family gathering without her. While our family is together, we schedule a party to celebrate Carol's 69th birthday on April First.

It is wonderful to see the kids and grandkids, but I feel guilty for enjoying myself while Carol is home alone. It is only for a few hours, but in the last several months the only times we have been apart was either when she was in the hospital or when I have gone grocery shopping or made frequent trips to the drugstore. I have a ways to go before I am fully living in non-duality. Attaining my own standards of "good/bad" and "right/wrong" has been a lifetime struggle.

Later, as I return to listening to Carol Ruth, I learn an even more insidious way in which I act out duality: for many years I have been searching for my true "self" believing I can finally know the "real" me. But she, almost laughingly, comments, "As if the self is something one can hold on to, define and put into concrete." She perfectly describes my battle to rid myself of my "dark" anger and reflect only love. I often fail, she explains, because the more I struggle to be free of anger, the more I attract it into my life. It seems there is always another driver who cuts me off on the freeway or some other non-loving person to "make me angry," (as if a total stranger controlled my emotions). Just last week I yelled at an older man, in a wheelchair in the bicycle lane of a busy street, who berated me for coming too close to him. (In truth, we were both scared.) As I assessed my behavior, my first thought was "Why did I react that way? That isn't who I am." Unfortunately, it was "who I am," even though I believe "I am much better than that."

"Non-dualistically…the self cannot be defined, confirmed, confined, or put into solidarity under any conditions. Because—the self is constantly molding, shaping, consistently changing 'something' and will never allow itself to be grasped or held onto—we must instead give it up, rather than preserve it." [lxiii] Wow!! I am taken aback. I think I know myself pretty well and now she tells me my "self" is unknowable because it is constantly changing and reinventing its "self." I'll have to sit with that for a while.

Carol Ruth continues now as if directly addressing my present situation. We look at illness through a dualistic lens: it is better to be healthy and worse to be ill. For many religions, including Christianity, healing disease is an important tenet. I certainly asked all our friends and family to pray for God (however they define

It) to take away Carol's cancer. Carol Ruth is saying it is possible for me to accept Carol's cancer as God unfolding whether she is cured or not. Right now, I feel firmly attached to her being healed, although I've known since her diagnosis that she might not be. But Carol Ruth cautions that maintaining my "fixed position" could be "more difficult and dangerous over the long run than willingly becoming fluid, moving, and creative."[lxiv] Okay, I can release the disappointment of Thanksgiving with our family and a Christmas gathering without Carol. And I accept the "is-ness" that Carol's cancer could be fatal, but I am committed to doing everything I can to help her heal from it and live. Is this dualistic thinking?

With the new year, Carol and I start a new round of Cribbage for "The Championship of the Whole World," one in which "chemo-brain" won't affect the outcome. We, also, begin reassessing our life and thinking what our "new normal" might look like. We had over-optimistically (and somewhat naively) believed she would feel well enough to return to her psychotherapy practice by now. Not only is she not ready to return, but, for the first time she is questioning whether she wants to resume marriage and family counseling at all. This is huge! Carol has long considered her psychotherapy practice as doing God's work. For the 25 years that I have known her, she has said she would continue her work in some capacity for the rest of her life. Cancer causes us to rethink our lives. Is this God unfolding?

In her lesson on non-duality, Carol Ruth quoted Luke 11:34-35 to illustrate a non-dualistic interpretation of this familiar passage: "Your eye is the lamp of your body; when your eye is sound, your whole body is full of light; but when it is not sound, your body is full of darkness. Therefore, be careful lest the light in you be darkness. If then your whole body is full of light, having no part dark, it will be wholly bright, as when a lamp with its rays gives you light."

Traditionally, dualistically, I have wanted my eye to be "sound," so I tried to fill my life with light by thinking pure thoughts, being kind to my neighbors, going to church, and doing what good Christians do. Carol Ruth proposes, "What if soundness of the eye is only to see what is?" Although light is often seen as the opposite of dark, she suggests there is another aspect within, "one we could call bright—one that…as a single eye … sees both light and dark without preference. The eye only has to be single." She continues, "What if the only darkness is the assumption that you are in darkness, which is the subtle belief that you think you know what is right or wrong—and even that is a part of the design of your process because it is even a part of the whole for you to have that question. Which means you cannot ever be not in God." [lxv] If I interpret this correctly, Carol Ruth is saying that a "sound eye" sees "what is" and the Truth of "what is" is that God is everywhere present. God is always present within me, even in my erroneous thought that I am separate from God. I have to sit with this for a while and let her words soak in and then percolate up from inside me.

As I'm considering this profound idea, I am aware of another unexpected development. Cancer has a profound psychological impact on the patient and the family. Even the word "cancer" creates a fear reaction in most people, including me and Carol Martha. Carol is a strong, self-confident, self-sufficient woman, but the cancer has shaken her belief in her abilities. Ordinary events, such as driving to the drug store, now seem daunting and require courage. The completion of each new/old task is cause for celebration. She is a new woman relearning to spread her wings and fly as she did before.

I read a newspaper article yesterday stating the psychological community is expanding its definition of posttraumatic stress to include the persistent effects of a serious illness or accident. I wanted to smack my forehead and go "Duh!" Everyone in the world must have realized this except me. Ovarian cancer is a deadly disease and certainly as much a threat as someone shooting at you and, therefore, capable of producing similar after-effects. I consider myself to be fairly intelligent, but sometimes I am amazed at how unaware I can be. Of course Carol is experiencing psychological effects.

I am beginning to feel this post-chemotherapy stage of recovery is more difficult psychologically than either the surgery or the chemotherapy itself. She doesn't suffer nearly the physical pain now, but our lives lack the strict regimen of that period. During chemo, every

Monday we went for lab tests, every third Monday the test included the CA-125 and that day we saw Doctor D'Andre. The following day Carol had chemo, followed on Wednesday by a Neulasta shot if needed. We knew Carol's worst day would be the day following a Neulasta shot. Then she would slowly begin to feel better. Our lives revolved around her chemo schedule. Chemotherapy provided our life structure for several months. Now that structure no longer exists and we can't get back to the life we had before.

Our friend Cass, a breast cancer survivor, was right when she said, "Your life will never be the same." We are still struggling to find our new "normal life." At the same time, I know "this is our 'normal life'."

I turn once again to Carol Ruth to learn more about non-duality. Using physics to support her point, she explains that for centuries our science, belief structure, legal system, psychology and spiritual beliefs have been based on Isaac Newton's system of physics that said objects we observe are outside ourselves and innately separate. In the early 1900s, Werner Heisenberg theorized there is "no reality outside of us—there is only the reality that is inside us and that reality sees all as it is, knows all as it is, and perceives all as it is." Heisenberg realized that "the minute an object is determined as a separate reality it is being formed by the consciousness looking at it." So there is nothing to get straight, "the internal consciousness sees reality [as] both right and wrong, good and bad, in its own way...It is what it is. There is no right or wrong out there—there is no out there—it is in you."[lxvi] Carol Ruth adds that "what is" also includes judgment. The "single eye" does not try to eliminate or condemn judgment, it just sees it for "what it is." "If you enter into the non-dualistic world, then you enter into a world where there is both good and bad, right and wrong, and there is some 'as well' (which I have come to see as accepting everything as it is) that wraps it. If you live in this concept, you do not live in an either/or world, you live in an 'as well' world."[lxvii]

As Valentine's Day approaches, Carol and I have much to celebrate: she continues to grow stronger, it is our twenty-second wedding anniversary, and we're having our first dinner date since her surgery. This is her first occasion to "get dressed up" and wear lipstick and make-up. She looks beautiful. Dinner at Scott's, a local restaurant, is wonderful. We eat slowly savoring every bite and every moment. Neither Carol nor I can stop smiling. Looking across the table at my beautiful wife, I realize how truly blessed I am. The perceptive server intuits that it is our anniversary and completes our dinner with a special dessert and her congratulations. The experience of these past months has deepened our love and drawn us even closer than we were before. In that way, the cancer has brought a gift. Aha, this is a non-dualistic awareness.

Continuing my look at non-duality, I watch the video of a later lesson entitled "Is Anything Right or Wrong or More Real than Anything Else?" Carol Ruth uses a green bug landing on her finger to illustrate this complex concept. The bug landing is a simple event (first dimension). But immediately her consciousness interprets the incident dualistically as "good" or "bad" and decides whether to knock the bug off her finger or let it stay (second dimension). She also recognizes that the bug is participating in the event whichever way she reacts (third dimension). Then she becomes aware that deep within her consciousness a "watcher" observes the event (fourth dimension). Finally a higher Universal or God consciousness views the entire scenario, sees the bug landing, observes the judgment that deems the incident right or wrong, knows that both the bug and the body on which it lands are participating, and watches the "watcher" (fifth dimension). This God consciousness knows that all parts are intended and nothing can be wrong, including killing the bug.[lxviii]

To make her message more relevant and more startling, she next proposes "a rape occurs." Again she calls it a "simple event" (first dimension). Our minds and our legal systems quickly label the event as "bad" - a criminal act - and we move to take care of the victim and punish the perpetrator (second dimension). We also recognize that the rape affects both the victim and the rapist at a level deeper than either can perceive (third dimension). Carol Ruth suggests the larger body on which the rape occurs is the "body of humanity" and it happens inside all of us, "nothing goes unfelt or unknown in the total human consciousness" (fourth dimension). Behind that is a deeper consciousness that "knows all levels are so." This God consciousness sees the rape take place, hears the statements of right or wrong, knows there is some divine intention (whether conscious or not), is aware of impact on the entire body of humanity, and, at a deeper level, knows all these dimensions are happening at the same instant, in the same place, and "nothing can be wrong." To emphasize her point she added, "If I should get raped or killed there would be some knowing in me that there is some divine intention deeper than my mind which I cannot figure out—life is not always fair; it does not always add up, figure out or work as we would have it, nor does it make sense or justify."[lxix] For nearly twenty-five years I have replayed this last statement in my head pondering if she had a premonition and was preparing us for her death, which came just a few weeks later.

Using Carol Ruth's line of reasoning, Carol's cancer could be seen as a "simple event," (first dimension) one that we judged "bad" and immediately sought help to get rid of it (second dimension). This event affected both Carol and me at a level deeper than either of us could perceive (third dimension). Inside each of us, a "watcher" observed the event (fourth dimension). And, above it all, God viewed the entire set of events knowing the cancer, the treatment, and the recovery were all intended and "nothing could be wrong" (fifth dimension). That is hard to take in. My first impulse is to ask, "Why?" But I know the answer is, "It just is!" I'll have to work with this for a while before it feels true to me.

The First of April soon arrives and our entire family gathers at our home for Carol's birthday. This is the first time we have all been together since our son and daughter-in-law's party just before Carol's surgery. She and our grandchildren have not seen each other for nearly a year. Throughout the day it seems there is always a child or grandchild with their arms around her. We have a couple of Carol's favorite treats: a huge "sushi boat" from the Blue Nami and a special Mirabel's chocolate birthday cake. I kidded Carol that the cake she selected looks like a wedding cake, but she said, "I don't care. I like it and that is the one I want." Everyone is having a wonderful time, especially Carol. It is cause for celebration. Family photographer, Granddaughter Aidan, takes lots of pictures, including shots of all of us together. It is a special day for everyone, with smiles and tears all around.

I have come to realize that daily life is the perfect classroom for spiritual lessons. Last Monday evening, just a few days after the birthday party, several men at my men's group meeting spoke of their fears. Listening, I found myself saying internally, "I am not afraid of that. Nor am I afraid of that." I could not relate to any of their fears. That left me with the question, "What am I afraid of?" I finally concluded, "I am afraid Carol's cancer will come back." Today, Friday, Greg and I had lunch and I shared with him my experience on Monday evening and the fear I did have.

When I arrive home, about 30 minutes later, Carol immediately informs me that she has a doctor's appointment in an hour. "Something in my abdomen doesn't feel right. I am afraid the cancer has come back." After a brief discussion, Doctor Spinelli refers us for a CT scan this afternoon. The scan goes smoothly, but, since it is Friday, there will no results until late Monday afternoon or Tuesday. This gives us the entire weekend to discuss "what ifs" and for me to confront my fear.

Carol has said repeatedly that she will not undergo chemotherapy again. It was too painful and too debilitating. I have doubted if I had the internal strength to repeat what has been one of the most difficult experiences of my life. The weekend wait allows plenty of time to talk and simply be present together. By Monday she decides that she can endure another round of chemotherapy if the cancer has returned. I know that I can be there again to love and support her. Life gave me an immediate opportunity to confront my greatest fear and I now can release that knowing I could face it if need be.

The CT scan results come back negative for cancer, but positive for two hernias. A few days later, Doctor Beneke explains hernias are common for ovarian cancer patients. The need for immediate chemotherapy can interfere with the healing of the surgery incision, resulting in hernias along the incision line. He recommends a rather simple surgery to repair the hernias, but says it is not absolutely necessary. The decision is Carol's. She opts for the surgery. Explaining the procedure, he explains he will reopen the incision line, insert a "mesh" material to reinforce the larger hernia site and close the smaller one with dissolvable sutures. She and Doctor Beneke agree it should be before the anniversary of her cancer surgery, so all the "bad stuff" can be confined to the same 12-month period.

The day of surgery is, as Yogi Berra said, "Déjà vu all over again." Both Carol and I relive last year's events as we enter the hospital, check in, take the elevator up to pre-op, and spend the time waiting for her to be wheeled into surgery. But, we reassure each other, "this is different," "this is a simple hernia surgery," "this will go quickly and you can begin healing immediately, there will be no chemotherapy after this surgery." The surgery does go quickly and as planned and Carol is soon in her room, two doors down the hall from the room she had last year. Another gift in the midst of pain, Carol's favorite nurse Maria, the "angel-of-mercy," is on duty. Two days later Carol is recovering at home.

Before this surgery, Carol talked with our daughter Sue, who had hernia surgery a couple years ago. Sue described the "mesh" material as resembling the webbing used for lawn-chairs. We all laughed at the thought. After surgery Carol dreamed she visited Doctor Beneke for her surgery follow-up appointment, when he said, "Many transplant patients want to meet the transplant donor. Would you like to meet the lawn-chair that donated the material for your surgery?" Carol, in the dream, replied, "I would and I wonder if it is related to the chair that donated material for my daughter's surgery." She had to share the dream with Doctor Beneke at her scheduled appointment and we all shared a laugh that made me realize how very different this moment is from last year's surgery follow-up appointment.

As I study non-duality and Carol Martha and I discuss it, I am beginning to understand this is the key to dealing with Carol's cancer. We recognize chemotherapy as the perfect analogy for non-duality. Chemo gives life by killing the cancer cells. During chemotherapy, Carol, surrounded by more love than she had ever felt, received an infusion of poison from a compassionate nurse. This life-threatening disease was the vehicle for a great outpouring of love and compassion from around the world. We are constantly surrounded by loving kindness from family, friends and complete strangers. We can feel our "oneness" with everyone.

"Why did Carol, who was doing God's work, get cancer?" is still a useless question for me. It just is. Why was Carol Ruth Knox, another woman doing God's work, murdered? I don't know. It just happened. How can I live my life non-dualistically, seeing God in everything, even Carol's cancer, knowing we are all one, while also seeing war, violence, famine and disaster? How can I live a non-dualistic life in a dualistic world? I think Ram Dass said it best, "The simple answer is that you do everything in the moment as if it had infinite meaning knowing full well it has absolutely none."[lxx]

But the key, for me, is even more basic. The late James Dillet Freeman, brilliant and beloved Unity author and poet, wrote "A Prayer of Protection," which concludes "wherever I am God is." I have recited this prayer hundreds, perhaps thousands, of times without truly considering the truth in this.

For my birthday, Carol and I spend the day at Stinson Beach. Sitting on my favorite rock, in my favorite spot, on my favorite beach, I suddenly realized the awesomeness of this statement.

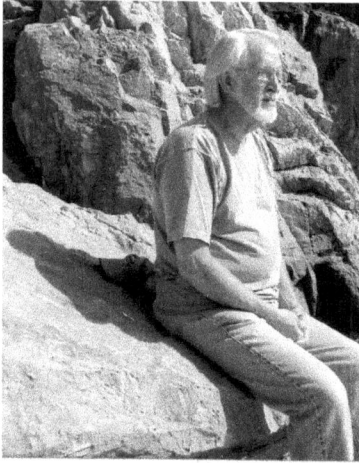

Coy at Stinson Beach - 2009

That is the answer to everything. My search for the "right way" to pray, to meditate, or to find the path to God's consciousness is as silly as the teenage Coy trying to find the correct way living a perfect life sixty years ago and presumes I am so brilliant that of the six billion plus people on the planet, I can figure out the correct answer to one of man's most profound questions. If God is "everywhere present," then God is present in me and all around me right now. Then I am permanently in God and God in me. When I bring my authentic self to God, God knows my heart and knows my desire to be in relationship, so there is no way that I can *not* "pray right," "meditate right," or can be disconnected from

God. God is present with Carol Ruth and was present when she died. God is also "everywhere present" in and around my wife Carol. God obviously must be in her cancer, too. God has not revealed to either her or me what this means yet. Maybe there is no deeper meaning, and I can accept that, too.

Wherever I am, God is.

God is right here, right now.

Nearer than my hands and feet,

Within my every breath and heartbeat,

God is,

God is

As I reflect over this past year and my efforts to deepen my spiritual process and to "see God in Carol's cancer," I chuckled to myself. I am back where I started, I have come full circle. I have to admit, though, I understand the circle a little better now. "Being consciously present" is my best way to participate in life. "Letting everything be as it is" is my only choice. To resist that is as silly as saying, "I won't accept that it is raining today." "Letting everything be as it is" is "coming from my heart and not my head." It is living in "Non-duality", which is also releasing a need for control and resting in "vehicle" in Carol Ruth's "victim/victor/vehicle." It is all One. This is The Dhance.

Chapter 7 - The Dhance

Life is not meant to be easy; life is meant to be great!

- James Dillet Freeman

And now I'm glad I didn't know
The way it all would end the way it all would go
Our lives are better left to chance
I could have missed the pain
But I'd of had to miss the dance.

- "The Dance," by Garth Brooks

Life continues to teach me that my greatest spiritual gifts come wrapped in my most difficult experiences. I read James Freeman's quote more than thirty years ago and it has given me courage to confront the challenges that have come to me. Some people, perhaps, do not need a cosmic two-by-four whack to awaken, but I haven't developed the skill to learn the easy way. This past year once again provided me with both the pain and the dance.

Carol Ruth often describes life as a dance, which she pronounces "dhance." She carefully differentiates dhance from recreational dancing by referring to Soren

Kierkegaard's description of living life as the dancer's leap. "It is supposed to be the most difficult task for a dancer to leap into a definite posture in such a way that there is not a second when he is grasping after the posture, but by the leap itself he stands fixed in that posture. Perhaps no dancer can do it—that is what the [person of true faith] does."[lxxi]

Most people are wallflowers, who sit along the wall and don't join in because they are afraid they will fall down. A person of true faith is a dancer, willing to fall, but even in the fall he/she is not "ungraceful to behold." The dancer is able to fall in such a way that it looks like they are "standing and walking to transform the leap of life into a walk, absolutely to express the sublime in the pedestrian."[lxxii]

Ram Dass, on the other hand, describes the "dhance" as a "cosmic giggle," which he identifies with his guru, Maharji. This giggle is "not of this world," but a "cosmic chuckle, the delight for the fun of it all. [Mahariji's] giggle was from the place that gives us the term 'lila,' the divine dance of life."[lxxiii]

I love both these images. If I am to dhance, Carol Ruth says I must move forward, without expecting a desired result; and yet the expectation of something helps me move forward. This, she calls, the "activity of God." God nudges me along by instilling an indwelling hunger into my soul, an insatiable hunger to stand in God's presence, while God, at the same time, desires my soul to be present with Him. "It is a [dhance] which humanity agrees to dance with God—a dance undertaken without promise or hope; yet each person knows that the dance will end in unification."[lxxiv]

This past year has been a classic lesson in non-duality in the midst of extremes as I strive to see the oneness that exists in "what is". It was and continues to be one of the hardest and most painful and at the same time one of the most joyous and profound times of my life. If life is a classroom, I've just completed graduate school and this book is my dissertation. Having the opportunity to face my greatest fear of her cancer returning convinced me I'm stronger than I previously thought. I know my perspective would be different, if Carol's cancer had been terminal. I believe, however, I would have still written a similar account of this time together, but I could not have written it this soon. I would have had to wait until the pain eased a bit.

As I acknowledged earlier, our friend Cass's prediction that our lives would never be the same is absolutely true. I know I will never be the person I was before. Fortunately I recognized almost immediately that I am not in charge and I could not heal Carol. What I could do was be consciously present with her. This, she later confirmed, was what she needed most. This has carried over and I now accept that God is in charge of my life and all I need to do is be consciously present in it. This, to me, is "being in the world and not of it."

Also, I have long envied men who write songs for their lovers or build houses for them. But the "song" I wrote and the "home we built" was one of being consciously present. Thus, by being consciously-with Carol, I could give her a far greater gift: the love, support and presence she needed to heal. This also allowed us to attend to what is most important in our lives: our love for each other, which deepen as we confronted her cancer together. I envy the song-writers and the builders no more.

The loving kindness that surrounded us throughout this year, from family, friends and the medical and support staff of Sutter Hospital, renewed my faith in humanity. People around the globe of various faiths, some of whom we don't even know, held Carol in prayer and love. She felt lifted up, supported and loved, and this had a profound impact on her healing. This convinced me that we are all one and living in a loving world. Truly, we are "all in this together."

Coming to understand that God is always present, even in the midst of cancer, has helped me accept "this is what is." From that position I see more clearly "what is given to me" to do next. Recognizing God as omnipresence assures me that my sincere prayers and meditations are connecting with that Universal Presence. I don't have to "know how to do it right," I can never do it wrong. In fact, trying to learn the "right way" to pray or meditate is an exercise to satisfy my ego, which can never succeed. I don't need the great mystical experience the saints often describe. I can now rest in God instead of seeking God. I simply open my eyes, ears and heart to what is around me. God is present right here, right now, in the sun and the rain, in the sea and the desert, in the flowers and the weeds, in the faces of the children and the ancients, in healing and sickness, and in Carol's cancer and in her recovery. This realization has brought more peace into my life.

Believing in God's omnipresence moves me to a deeper understanding of non-duality. With God as the only presence, nothing can be separate from God. I don't have to ask "why did God let Carol get cancer?" or "why would God let someone kill Carol Ruth?" I simply need to accept "what is": Carol had cancer and Carol Ruth was killed. God was and continues to be present in both. Accepting "what is," is moving to non-duality. Living non-dualistically in a dualistic world is "The Dhance."

While Carol Ruth quotes Kierkegaard, I love country-western philosopher Garth Brooks' lyrics in "The Dance." Indeed, if I had known in advance of the pain Carol and I would confront, I would have tried to avoid it. But then I would have missed The Dhance. When I consider how my life has unfolded in the past year, I realize I have often been Dhancing. When I agreed to "let everything be as it is," I was Dhancing. When I decided to simply be "consciously present" with Carol, I was Dhancing. When I refused to ask "Why?" and instead accepted "this is what is given me to do," I was Dhancing.

I came to fully understand The Dhance just over a year after Carol's surgery. Nearly two years earlier, while visiting her mother, Carol joined Kay and her friends for their weekly Tonk card game. During the game, Karleen, the hostess, mentioned she had trouble sleeping the night before. Carol responded that the moon had been full the previous night and she often had difficulty sleeping during the full moon. In jest, Carol continued, "What I do when I can't sleep during the full moon is take off all my clothes, put flowers in my hair, and dance naked in the moonlight." Five elderly mouths dropped open, with a unified, "No, you don't do that!" Staying in character, Carol replied, "I do, then I come back inside and sleep like a baby." This has been a running joke with these women every time they have seen Carol since then.

There was a full moon on June 26, this year. Around midnight Carol and I sat watching television when she said, "I'm going to do it. I'm going to do what I said." Not knowing what she was referring to, I asked, "You're going to do what?" "Dance naked in the moonlight," she replied. "Give me five minutes and then look out on the deck." Five minutes later, I saw one of the most beautiful sights of my life, my sixty-nine-year-old wife, surgical scars and all, dancing naked under the full moon. That is The Dhance.

Indeed, "life is not meant to be easy; life is meant to be [and is] great."

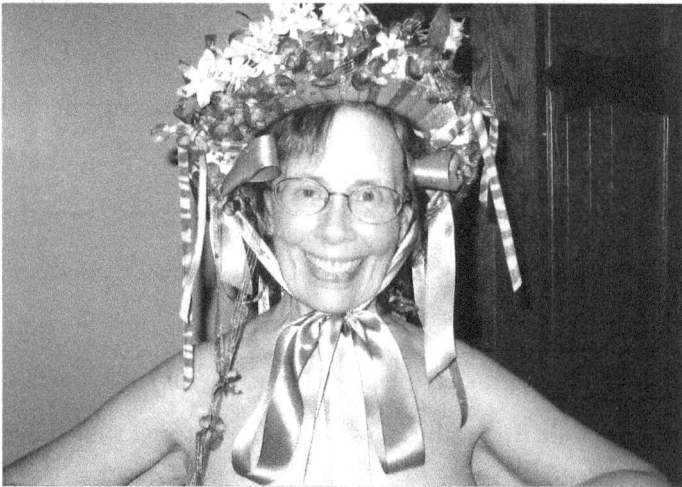

Carol Martha Ready to Dhance in the Moonlight

Epilogue
by Carol Martha

My mother asks, "When is your next check-up?" I am aware that although it is only one month away, I am calm, without the anticipatory anxiety that has preceded each follow-up appointment since remission. I also am noticing now the calm, yet joyful excitement of Christmas coming—the house to decorate, tree to trim, food to cook, to host our Circle of Light party. The "Circle of Light" is when we come together with friends and family to light candles to honor, bless, give thanks and raise hope for our Circle, our community, our nation and the world beyond.

What is the lightness and inner peace I feel? Is it just time and acceptance of living with my experience with cancer or is it something more?

Three nights ago Coy and I were talking after he had read a rewrite of Chapter Two. He has used me for reflection and feedback from the first days of gestation, when we talked of a book needing to be born about Carol Ruth's teachings as applications for living. The gestation has taken more than ten years now.

Throughout our relationship, I have felt a spiritual, physical magnetic pull to live this chapter of my life with this man. I fancied myself as his muse. My personal philosophy has always been that everything that has happened before in my life leads me to the present moment. As a working psychotherapist I was able to live this philosophy and bring not only my education but my life wisdom to the moments spent with clients. I could see, "Oh, that's why I had to go through that. Now I can use that wisdom with the person before me." This is how I believed I was manifesting Carol Ruth's teaching of moving from Victim—to Victor—to Vehicle.

To my great frustration, my life chapter called "Cancer: My Dark Night and What Follows" had held little meaning for me. I didn't "get it." I experienced regressing from Vehicle to Victim and back to Victor as I saw that for now at least I was surviving. But what of this experience was bringing me to Vehicle, to being the messenger of my experience as before?

Three nights ago, "I got it." Being the Vehicle

doesn't always mean I am doing the driving. My chapter called "Cancer: My Dark Night and What Follows" stimulated my husband's writing of this book, shifting the focus from intellectual teaching to experiential meaningfulness. Although the trappings of my day-to-day life seem to have dwindled to less contact with the community, the "muse" lives on. Each experience in life offers an opportunity to take us deeper in spiritual understanding. Carol Ruth used to say, as a way of synthesizing non-duality into daily living, "And this, too, and this, too, and this, too. . . ."

This, too, "Cancer: My Dark Night and What Follows," floats into place continuing the pattern of all things leading to this present moment. Thank you, Coy, for letting me be the muse and giving my life ongoing meaning.

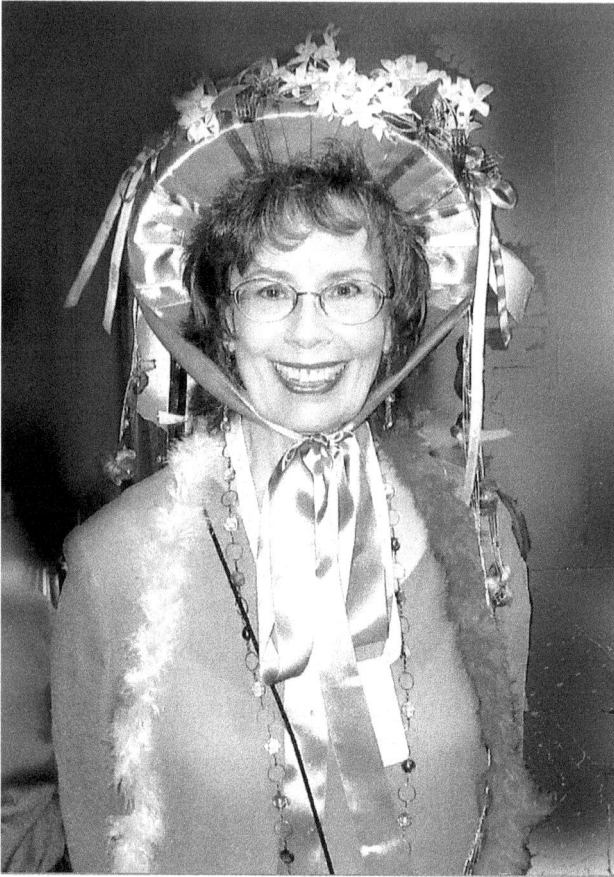

Carol In Her Dhancing Flowers

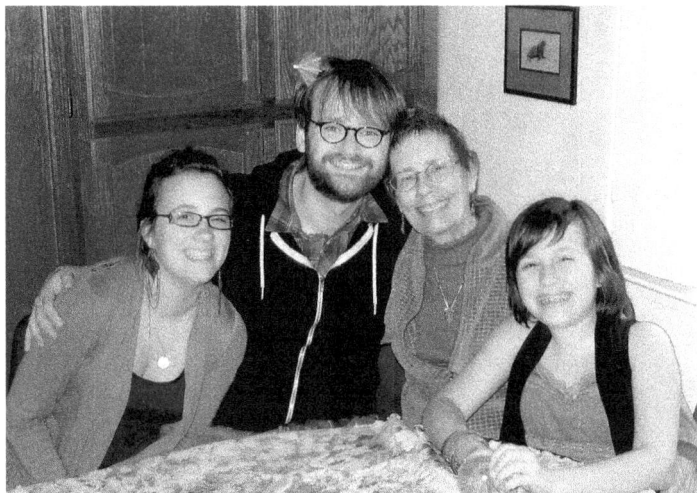

Carol with Grandchildren Aidan, James, and Spencer at Carol's birthday - 2010

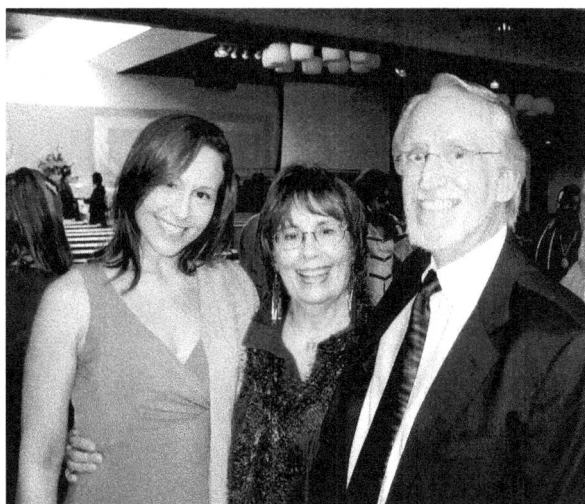

Daughter Susan, Carol, and Coy - 2007

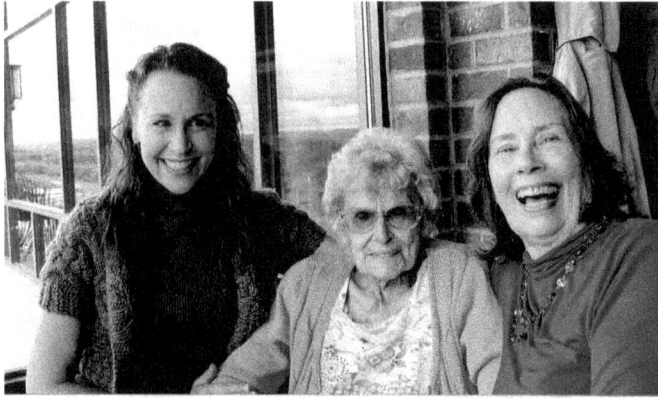

Daughter Susan, Mother Kay, and Carol - 2011

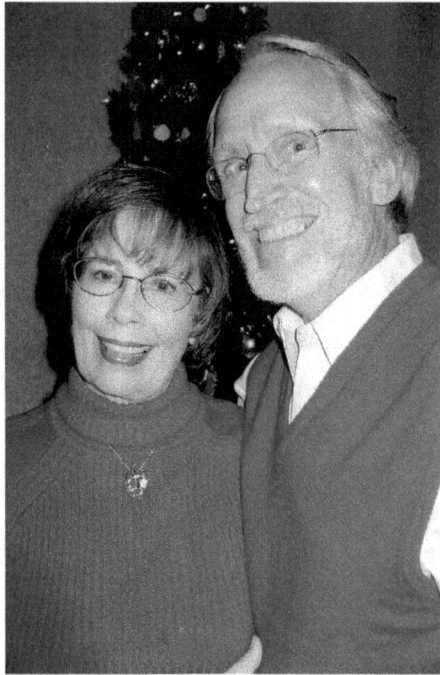

Carol and Coy - 2010

Process Chart

This diagram will assist in explaining the different layers as Carol Ruth perceived them in a person's growth and development. It gives a "feeling" for levels of soul evolution in what appears to be three stages.

There have, no doubt, been earlier ones that no longer can be seen as they have been lopped off in the evolutionary process. She had not experienced levels beyond the mystical, but sensed they were possible. Words defining each stage are listed parallel to each other.

Be careful of your individual response to the words as they have deeper and more complex meanings than their simple usage often denotes.

Process Chart		
Traditional (Victim)	First closet (Birth canal)	Metaphysical (Victor)
Unconscious		Conscious
Waiting		Doing/having
Physical		Emotional
Instinctual		Mental
1st chakra		2nd and 3rd chakra
No ego		Strong ego
Has no effect	Death of dependent Self	Karmic law
No choice		Choice
No will		Will
No control		Control/manipulation
Begging		Affirmation/denial
Irresponsibility		Responsibility

Process Chart	
Second closet (Birth canal)	**Mystical (Vehicle)**
	Consciously not conscious
	Being
	Spiritual
	Intuitive
4th chakra	5th through 7th chakra
	Egoless
Dark Night of the soul	Beyond Karmic
	Freedom from choice
Death of self	Divine will
	Give up control
	Ongoing prayer (grace)
	Available to respond

About the Author

Coy Cross is a well-respected author and speaker. He runs workshops which delve deeply into Rev Knox's teachings. Selected topics include: _The Dhance - A Caregiver's Search For Meaning_ and _I Let Everything Be As It Is_. Dr. Cross also gives Sunday Lessons at Unity Churches based on the mystical teachings of Rev. Knox especially as they relate to acceptance and transformation.

Other books by Dr. Coy F. Cross II include:

Lincoln's Man in Liverpool: Consul Dudley and the Legal Battle to Stop Confederate Warships (2007),

Justin Smith Morrill Father of the Land-Grant Colleges (1999),

From the Stone Age to the Space Age: a History of Beale AFB (1997),

Go West Young Man! Horace Greeley's Vision for America (1995),

and jointly authored by Roger D. Launius and Coy F. Cross II _MAC and the Legacy of the Berlin Airlift_

(Monograph of the Military Airlift Command, Office of History) (1989).

Dr. Cross has also edited Carol Ruth Knox's book, *Path of God* (2013).

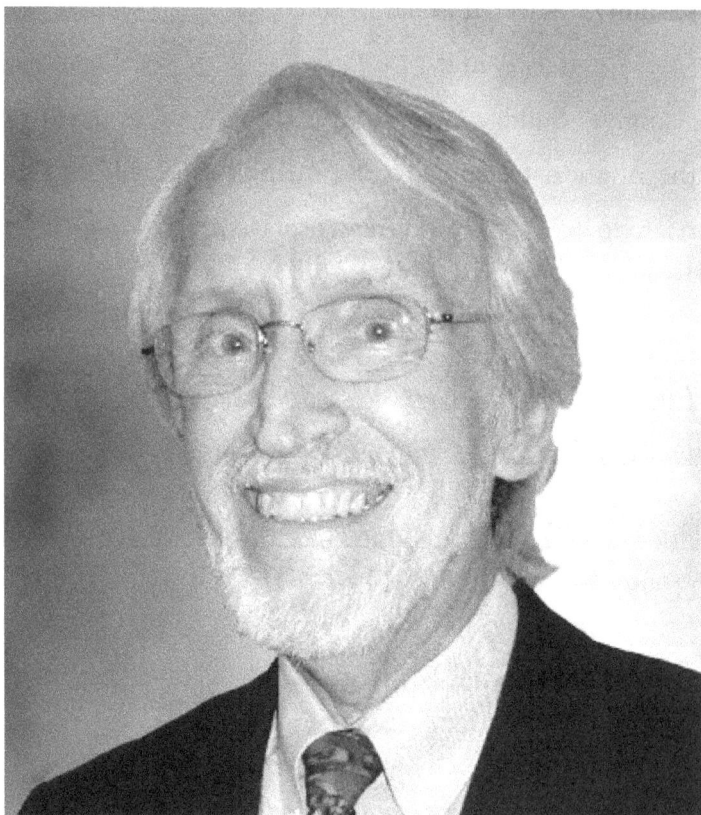

Author Coy F. Cross II

The Path of God, Edited By Coy F. Cross II

Explore THE PATH G OF with Rev. Carol Ruth Knox

Each Sunday Rev. Carol Ruth Knox shared how she encountered God that past week and she spoke about the lessons she learned in terms of quantum physics, philosophy, Eastern religions, and whatever subject caught her interest. Attendees left with helpful tools for their daily lives.

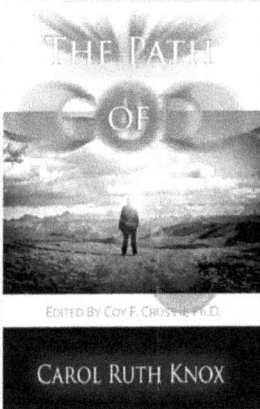

Her powerful and still-relevant messages resonate today and can help you achieve a life of meaning, of service and of spiritual mastery by embracing The Path of God.

EDITED BY COY F. CROSS II, Ph.D.

Available to conduct Sunday Service, 3-hour workshops Sunday afternoon, and Book Signings.

* $14.95
* softcover
* 244 pages

Endnotes

[i] Carol Ruth Knox, Sunday lesson, "Alternate Realities: Is anything right or wrong or more real than anything else?" 5Oct 86.

[ii] *Carol Ruth Knox, "Alternate Realities: Is anything right or wrong or more real than anything else?" Sunday Lesson, Oct 5, 1986.*

[iii] *Notes from "Lesson in Truth" class taught by Rev Jim Lee.*

[iv] *Fillmore, quoted in Freeman,* The Story of Unity, *194.*

[v] *Carol Ruth Knox,* Unity: A Spiritual Path *(Walnut Creek CA: Unity Center, 1984), 3-5, 6-7.*

[vi] *Knox,* Unity, *3-5.*

[vii] *Knox,* Unity, *12 & 16.*

[viii] *Knox,* Unity, *50.*

[ix] *Carol Ruth Knox, "And Where is the Passion in Spirituality?" Sunday Lesson, 13Jan85.*

[x] *Knox,* Unity, *52.*

[xi] *Interview with Carol Ruth Knox (interviewer unknown), 1986.*

[xii] *Ibid.*

[xiii] *Carol Ruth Knox,* The Incredible Journey *(Walnut Creek CA: Unity Center, 1984), 39-40.*

[xiv] *Carol Ruth Knox, "Must I lie down and be Tromped on to be Spiritual?" Sunday Lesson, 20Jan85.*

[xv] *Knox,* Unity, *40-41.*

[xvi] *Ibid, 41-42.*

[xvii] *Ibid, 42-46.*

[xviii] *Ibid, 52.*

[xix] *Ibid, 53-54.*

[xx] *Eric Butterworth,* Discover the Power Within You *(San Francisco: Harper, 1989), 105.*

[xxi] *Carol Ruth Knox, "The Path of Prayer," Sunday lesson, 9Mar86.*

[xxii] *Carol Ruth Knox, "Our Father, Who art in Heaven," Sunday lesson, 2 Jan 1978; "Give us This Day our Daily Bread and Forgive us our Debts as we also have Forgiven our Debtors,"*

Sunday lesson, 16 Jan 1978; "Leave us not in Temptation,"
Sunday lesson, 23 Jan 1978; "For Thine is the Kingdom and
the Power and the Glory Forever," Sunday lesson, 30Jan1978.

xxiii Carol Ruth Knox, "Black Magic," Sunday lesson, 31 Oct 76.

xxiv Carol Ruth Knox, "The Path of Prayer," Sunday lesson,
9Mar86.

xxv Carol Ruth Knox, "When you don't expect it, things go back and
forth between Terrific and Terrible," Sunday lesson, 15Sep85.

xxvi Carol Ruth Knox, "The Path of Prayer," Sunday lesson,
9Mar86.

xxvii Carol Ruth Knox, "When you don't expect it, things go back
and forth between Terrific and Terrible," Sunday lesson,
15Sep 85.

xxviii Carol Ruth Knox, "An Ancient Art of Prayer," Sunday lesson,
25 Jan 81.

xxix Carol Ruth Knox, "An Ancient Art of Prayer," Sunday lesson,
25 Jan 81; Carol Ruth Knox, "Lent Wings," Sunday lesson,
5Feb 78.

xxx Carol Ruth Knox, "An Ancient Art of Prayer," Sunday lesson,
25Jan 81.

xxxi Carol Ruth Knox, "An Ancient Art of Prayer," Sunday lesson,
25Jan 81.

xxxii Carol Ruth Knox, Meditation Workshop, October 1986.

xxxiii Charles Fillmore, The Essential Charles Fillmore, 36-37.

xxxiv Fillmore, Essential, 127.

xxxv Ibid, 128-29.

xxxvi Cady, Lessons in Truth, 105-110.

xxxvii Butterworth, The Universe is Calling, 75-77.

xxxviii Ibid, 78-81.

xxxix Joel S. Goldsmith, The Art of Meditation (San Francisco:
Harper and Row, Publishers, 1956), 13.

xl Joel S. Goldsmith, The Contemplative Life (Secaucus NJ: The
Citadel Press, 1963), 93.

xli Ibid., 95.

xlii Carol Ruth Knox, Meditation Workshop, October 1986.

xliii Ibid.

xliv Ibid.

xlv Ibid.

[xlvi] *Ibid.*

[xlvii] *CRK, "Prayer of the Heart" workshop, Mar84.*

[xlviii] *CRK dissertation, 34-35.*

[xlix] *CRK dissertation, 30.*

[l] *Joel S.* Goldsmith, Practicing the Presence: The Inspirational Guide to Regaining Meaning and a Sense of Purpose in Your Life *(San Francisco: Harper San Francisco, 1958), 9.*

[li] *Goldsmith,* Practicing the Presence, *96.*

[lii] *Goldsmith,* Practicing the Presence, *97.*

[liii] *CRK, Sunday message, "The Flame in the Heart," 24Oct 82.*

[liv] *CRK dissertation, 127.*

[lv] *CRK, "The Prayer of the Heart," workshop, Mar84.*

[lvi] *CRK, "The Prayer of the Heart," workshop, Mar84.*

[lvii] *CRK dissertation, 31.*

[lviii] *CRK dissertation, 127.*

[lix] *CRK, "The Prayer of the Heart," workshop, Mar84.*

[lx] *Jo Dunning quoting Carol Ruth Knox, Introduction to "The Path of Non-Duality," 23 Feb 86, reissued by Carol Ruth Knox Foundation, 1988.*

[lxi] *Carol Ruth Knox, Sunday lesson, "The Path of Non-Duality," 23Feb 86.*

[lxii] *Carol Ruth Knox, Sunday lesson, "The Path of Non-Duality," 23Feb 86.*

[lxiii] *Carol Ruth Knox, Sunday lesson, "The Path of Non-Duality," 23Feb 86.*

[lxiv] *Carol Ruth Knox, Sunday lesson, "The Path of Non-Duality," 23Feb 86.*

[lxv] *Carol Ruth Knox, Sunday lesson, "The Path of Non-Duality," 23Feb 86.*

[lxvi] *Carol Ruth Knox, Sunday lesson, "The Path of Non-Duality," 23Feb 86.*

[lxvii] *Carol Ruth Knox, Sunday lesson, "The Path of Non-Duality," 23Feb 86.*

[lxviii] *Carol Ruth Knox, Sunday lesson, "Alternate Realities: is anything right or wrong or more real than anything else?" 5Oct 86.*

[lxix] *Carol Ruth Knox, Sunday lesson, "Alternate Realities: is anything right or wrong or more real than anything else?" 5Oct 86.*

[lxx] *Quoted, Carol Ruth Knox, Sunday lesson, "The Path of Non-Duality," 23Feb 86.*

[lxxi] *Soren Kierkegaard,* Fear and Trembling and the Sickness Unto Death, *trans. Walter Lowrie (Princeton: Princeton University Press, 1941), 52.*

[lxxii] *Soren Kierkegaard,* Fear and Trembling and the Sickness Unto Death, *trans. Walter Lowrie (Princeton: Princeton University Press, 1941), 52.*

[lxxiii] *Ram Dass,* Journey of Awakening: A Meditator's Guidebook *(New York: Bantam Books, 1978), 203.*

[lxxiv] *Carol Ruth Knox, dissertation, 192.*